■THE■ HELP YOURSELF™ L♥VE YOURSELF

NonDiet WEIGHT-LOSS PLAN

Dr. Joel C. Robertson

OLIVER NELSON

THOMAS NELSON PUBLISHERS
Nashville

Published in Nashville, Tennessee, by Oliver-Nelson Books, a division of Thomas Nelson, Inc., Publishers, and distributed in Canada by Lawson Falle, Ltd., Cambridge, Ontario.

Unless otherwise noted, the Bible version used in this publication is THE NEW KING JAMES VERSION. Copyright © 1979, 1980, 1982, Thomas Nelson, Inc., Publishers. Scripture quotations noted TEV are from the *Good News Bible*—Old Testament: Copyright © American Bible Society 1976: New Testament: Copyright © American Bible Society 1966, 1971, 1976. Used by permission.

Printed in the United States.

Library of Congress Cataloging-in-Publication Data

Robertson, Joel C., 1952-
   The help yourself love yourself nondiet weight loss plan / Joel C. Robertson.
     p.   cm.
  ISBN 0-8407-9135-6
  1. Reducing. I. Title.
RM222.2.R59 1992
613.2'5—dc20   92-29491
                                     CIP

1 2 3 4 5 6 — 97 96 95 94 93 92

Dedication

This book is dedicated to my wife, Vickie, who continues to be supportive. She has made our home a haven and a relaxing environment that encourages, protects, and energizes us all.

To Nicole, Heidi, and Brooke, my three adorable daughters, for their ability to keep Daddy a daddy and not a professional.

To my parents, James and Evelyn Robertson, and my wife's parents, George and Arlene Leinberger, for giving me wisdom that comes from experiencing life.

And finally to Dennis Brown, whose friendship and wisdom I have appreciated. A truly successful and talented businessman, whose willingness to share himself and his faith inspires me and all who work with him at Diet Center, Inc.

I am truly a fortunate man to have these people in my life.

Contents

Acknowledgments

This book is the result of the talent and hard work of several individuals. I would like to thank them for their energy and insight in developing this book.

Thanks to Cecil Murphey, a true friend and a special writer, for his compassion and skills as a writer. Victor Oliver, a publisher who continues to impress me with his knowledge of people, insight, and consideration of others. Rose Marie Sroufe, administrative assistant at Oliver-Nelson, for responding to the many requests I make. Bruce Barbour, publisher at Thomas Nelson, for his encouragement and excitement about the project. Bob Zaloba, marketing director at Thomas Nelson, for his truly amazing talent at marketing a book. And Lila Empson, a talented, caring, and overall great editor to work with.

These people and the many patients I have met and interviewed have helped me develop this book so that you may help yourself.

Introduction

Telling you about the problem with my ponies may be the best way of explaining what this book is about. I own two Shetland ponies, and they have eight acres to run on. Also on those eight acres, I have a nice barn that measures twelve feet by twenty feet.

Although the situation had been going on for some time, I had not paid much attention to it. Then one morning I walked around while sipping my second cup of coffee, relaxing, and enjoying the beginning of a new day. One of the ponies was more than two hundred yards from the barn. She grazed along like any normal animal. Suddenly, her tail went up. She turned around and raced for the barn as if a hunter were chasing her. She didn't stop until she was inside the barn. Just then I realized why she ran into the barn.

"With all that land for the ponies' use," I said disgustedly, even though no one was with me, "where do the ponies leave their manure? Why don't they use the field like other animals? Why do they have to tear back into the barn every time?"

Day after day, I watched both horses rush back to the barn every time they wanted to eliminate. The more I thought about their behavior, the more personally I took their actions. *I* was the one who had to clean up their mess.

In the field, the manure would benefit the soil by helping to fertilize it. Besides, I wouldn't have to deal with it. But because they insisted on going inside my barn, I was forced to do something to change the situation.

Because of my nature, I wanted to solve the problem right then—not later, not on Saturday morning or Thursday afternoon. I burst into a furor of activity. Grabbing the pitchfork, I decided how to clean it up. In a couple of minutes, I'd be rid of the large pile. That's when I learned my first lesson.

I realized that if I tried to do it all in one motion—pushing

1

the pitchfork down to the bottom of the pile and pulling up as hard as I could—I would end up face down in the manure. The big load was too heavy for me. So I reasoned that if I started at the top of the pile, I could take out small loads, one at a time. It was a slow procedure, but eventually, I got rid of all of it. The first lesson I learned was that cleaning up required a steady, methodical solution with no shortcuts.

Then I learned a second lesson: If I didn't want more messes in my barn, all I had to do was close the barn door and keep it closed. If I wanted to be free from the unpleasant task of cleaning up after the horses, all I had to learn was how to close the door. Only then could I say to myself, "The barn is finally clean for good. From now on, I'm keeping the door closed so the horses won't come in here again." Then I could feel peaceful and enjoy my clean barn, and my horses could fertilize up to eight acres of grassy field.

That's exactly what I did: I closed the door.

The two lessons I learned actually explain the goal and purpose of this book. I want to help you use sensible, methodical ways to clean up your addictive behavior. First, I'll help you get rid of your habitual, ongoing dieting, your chronic-and-constant thinking about food. I'm going to help you take it one pitchfork load at a time. Each little pitchforkful takes you closer and closer to cleaning it all up. Then I'll help you do the second thing: You'll learn to close the barn door and keep it closed.

To help you get your first load on the pitchfork, I want you to know one important fact right now: *The Help Yourself Love Yourself Nondiet Weight Loss Plan* is *not* a diet book—just as the name says. From these pages, you will *not* learn

- about a breakthrough miracle diet.
- how to cut calories.
- new methods to cut your fat intake.
- fifteen ways to trim your weight by fifteen pounds in fifteen days.

This book is for those of you who have tried the diets. You can describe every diet invented during the past few years. You hear yourself saying to others such things as:

- "I've been on every diet in the world, and I'm still too heavy."
- "I can lose weight on any diet I try, but then I always gain it back again—that and more."
- "I have three sizes—skinny, normal, and big—but most of the time I'm big."
- "I've lost 200 pounds in the last several years. I've also gained 212 pounds."

I'm not offering you a diet plan, although I will offer you suggestions on better eating habits and on particular foods that will help you alter your moods. This book is dedicated to those people who have lost the extra pounds and now struggle to keep the weight off.

I want to stress this point: You don't need this book to lose weight. Many different diet plans, programs, and organizations can help you drop the pounds. You can try Overeaters Anonymous or programs such as Diet Centers, or you can follow diets laid out in the latest diet books on the bookstore shelves. You can lose weight with over-the-counter products, physicians' prescribed diets, or franchised weight management programs. (You should be aware that some of these approaches are healthier than others. Consideration of that subject, however, is not within the scope of this book.)

Yet if you're a regular, compulsive dieter, you know immediately that you're back inside the barn, cleaning up the mess you've made. You've cleaned up a dozen times, but the horses keep coming back. You don't know how to shut the barn door. Or to state the problem from your perspective, the question is, How do I keep the weight off?

I am going to teach you how to take one pitchfork load at a time. Among other things, throughout this book, I am going to give you self-affirmation statements, which I call vital facts. They are vital in the sense that it is crucial for you to acknowledge them as true. If you acknowledge them as true—no matter how unpleasant they may sound at first—you are already on your way to keeping the weight off.

Read each affirmation aloud at least six times a day. As you speak the words and hear yourself say them, think of yourself lifting one small load out of the pile.

♥ ♥ ♥

A vital fact about myself: I have a
problem with food.

♥ ♥ ♥

(By the time you finish this book, you will no longer need to
say that you have a problem with food. Once you have learned
to close the door, you will eliminate your problem.)

Please don't laugh at this statement. Thousands of people
deny they have a problem. Or they explain it away by saying
things such as:

- "My parents overfed me."
- "My friends insist, 'Just one more. This little bit
  won't hurt you.'"
- "I say to my husband (or wife), 'You make me so
  angry. That's why I eat so much.'"
- "The media throw food ads at me every time I watch
  TV, listen to the radio, or read a magazine. No
  wonder I eat too much."

Like them, you also may have learned to offer excuses to
yourself. Those excuses are usually a form of denial. You've
never faced the first real issue: You have a problem with food.

The truth is, you are *dependent* on food. I don't mean that
you need food to live. You depend on food for needs other than
nutrition and health. You are food dependent.

If you're like millions of others, you don't understand what
the term *dependency* means. I use the word to mean the same
thing as *addiction*. I don't distinguish between them because
both terms say that you need something

- to make you feel all right.
- to help you function properly.
- to take away your loneliness.
- to ease your inner pain.
- to give you a sense of self-worth.

When you need "something" to make you feel good—whether

it's food, alcohol, sex, gambling, work, or nicotine—you are *dependent. You are addicted.*

But you don't have to remain helpless and powerless. My purpose in writing is to tell you that you can be free forever. However, between your enslavement to food and your victory, you will have to take many steps. And you can take them. Others have done it. So can you.

I hope you'll accept your dependency and determine to change. Admitting you have a problem is important for your motivation to change. If your goal is not to overeat again, you have to face the reality of your food dependency.

If you're really bold and ready to face a challenge, you can change vital fact number one to read:

❤ ❤ ❤

A vital fact about myself: I am addicted to overeating.

❤ ❤ ❤

At several points in this book, I use material adapted from one of my previous books, *Help Yourself.* My purpose in doing so is to make it possible for you to address your food-dependency issues with *The Help Yourself Love Yourself Nondiet Weight Loss Plan* alone. Instead of assuming that you are familiar with some key definitions and explanations from *Help Yourself,* I repeat them here. You will then be able to understand the application of those principles to recovery from food dependency. I hope you find this approach helpful.

1

♥

But Why?

"I don't just *like* food," she said. "I have an ongoing affair with food. Food is on my mind all the time. I'm constantly thinking of what I have just eaten or when I'm going to eat next."

The thirty-year-old woman had a problem with food. She was honest enough to tell me how pervasive the matter of food was to her. She was a compulsive purger. She ate until she felt stuffed and then hurried to a bathroom to induce vomiting.

Even though your battle with food may not be this serious and compulsive, your situation is something you have to face. The fact that you're reading this book implies that you are at least interested enough to consider you might have a problem with food dependency. That's the first step.

As you read this book, I hope you'll also be able to admit, "Yes, I do have a problem. And I want help." When you reach that stage, you are ready to face yourself and begin working toward victory.

For years you may have felt anger for constantly struggling over food and your eating patterns, especially when you see others who gorge themselves and never seem to gain a pound. You've asked yourself hundreds of times,

- Why me?
- Why do *I* have a problem with food?
- Why is food so important in my life?
- Why can't I control my appetite?

- Why do I constantly overeat or else feel such a fear
  that I will overeat?

The reasons vary, of course. In the chapters ahead, I'll help
you see the cause of your eating problems. From that insight,
you can start taking steps to correct your addictive behavior.

First, let's look at who you are now. You may already have
partial explanations for your eating problems. Perhaps one of
these statements describes you:

- I'm under constant pressure (internal and exter-
  nal), so I eat to relieve the stress.
- I eat and eat and eat because I feel unloved, un-
  wanted, and misunderstood.
- I try hard, but I'm just not as good or as capable as
  I feel I have to be. So I eat.
- From childhood, whenever something was wrong, I
  learned that eating was a way to stop the deep hurt
  I was feeling.

Whatever the reason for your dependency on food, you are
now at the place in your life where you want to change. Maybe
you're so tormented you know you *have* to make a change. I'd
like you to pause and finish this sentence for yourself: I am
involved with (or addicted to or dependent on) food because...

Because the situation is complex, you may not be aware of
the reasons for your problem with food. The causes may be so
deep-seated, you don't recognize them. (I'll help you discover
those issues.)

Just admitting the problem isn't enough, either. Suppose
you attended one of my lectures, and I asked, "How many of
you want to stop overeating?" Would you raise your hand?
Probably you would.

Yet deep inside, a tiny voice would whisper to you, "I do
want to stop, but I also get a lot of pleasure from eating. I want
to stop, but at the same time, I don't really want to. I want to
stop gaining weight. I hate feeling flabby. Because I know I
need to stop overeating, I'm willing to do something. Yeah, but
I remember last time when..."

The voice says, "I want to change, but..."

If this voice sounds like the one that speaks to you, that's all right. That is where you are now. You've tried before and ended up frustrated and angry with yourself. You think of past failures. Because you let yourself down in the past, you're not sure you can handle another failure.

Perhaps you regularly make resolutions to eat only a certain amount. For instance, you decide to eat only one cookie and then stop. But you don't stop as you promised yourself. You eat until the bag is empty, your stomach is bloated, and you feel miserable. Then you hate yourself for being so weak-willed: "If only I had enough willpower, I could stop."

Your friends say, "Just stop. That's all you have to do. Push away from the table." The more they lecture, the worse you feel.

Maybe you experience a sense of loss, an undescribable fear that comes from giving up something that you don't want to give up. Perhaps you're in school, and you're having trouble with your grades. Eating relieves the pressure of having to compete. Or your on-the-job stress has gotten worse. Taking a few minutes out for a doughnut or a second sandwich eases the situation.

Whatever the pressure, I urge you not to direct your anger against yourself for being weak-willed. That isn't the center of the problem. You're concentrating on a perception and not on the cause.

Instead, think of what motivated you to read this book. You must have some level of motivation to have read even this far. You must have some desire to stop your compulsive overeating.

So why are you reading this book? Here are some possible answers from what others have told me when we've worked on their eating problems:

- "I'm filled with feelings of fear (or lack of self-confidence or a different emotion)."
- "I don't think I have a serious problem. A little bit of a problem, but nothing big. I'm just getting information."
- "I know I have to do something, but I'm afraid that I'll lose control (power) over my own life. That scares me."
- "I'm lonely because I don't have any close friends or relationships or those I have are falling apart."

- "I don't know the answer, but when I started feeling lonely (or whatever the feeling), I started becoming food dependent."

Your goal is to change your life. You want off the losing-gaining treadmill; you want to overcome your obsession with food. I want to point out six reasons for you to change.

1. You can have personal freedom

You will find freedom when you're not mastered by food. Whenever you feel you need to do something to feel better or you want to celebrate, you have this gnawing inside that says, "I've got to have food." Food controls you. You have no choice. No choice means no personal freedom. Personal freedom says, "I call the shots. I am in control of my life—and my eating."

2. You can have personal peace

Having personal peace enables you to say, "Sure, I've got hassles, but I also have a deep-seated inner tranquility." Right now you don't have that. You may be experiencing an emptiness inside, a void of some kind. It's empty even when your life is going smoothly. You may feel wonderful for a little while, but then the emptiness returns.

3. You can change for yourself

You need to want to be different for yourself. No longer content to fail, to quit, to run away from your food problem, you want your life to be different. You may even hear yourself saying, "This is something I'm doing for myself."

4. You can change because you love your family

Your family includes your spouse, parents, grandparents, siblings, and/or children. Although you need to look out for yourself, you are not living in isolation in the world. Your family members care—even if they don't know how to express it. When you help yourself, you're helping the entire family situation be healthier and happier. When you are the best you can be, you are also the best example you can be for them. Your good health and freedom from food dependency can shape the future of your family.

5. You can change to improve your health

I'm sure you want to live as long as you can continue to live a healthy life-style without disease and organ failures. As you probably know, obesity and other eating disorders contribute to many diseases, such as diabetes and heart problems. Once you make changes, you don't have fear that your life-style is contributing to these diseases.

6. You can change to maximize who you are

This reason is the important one. You are somebody special, even if you can't acknowledge it. You may not know what your specialness is because you've crowded your life with the issue of food. You can be tremendously rewarded by understanding that you're special.

As you read through this book, the most essential thing I can offer you is *hope*. Recovery is barely around the corner for you. Recovery is something that happens to people who want to change and who have enough information and skills to change. This opportunity to change is what I offer you in *The Help Yourself Love Yourself Nondiet Weight Loss Plan.*

♥ ♥ ♥

Before you read further, I want you to give careful consideration to any medical problems you may have. I'm going to identify specific exercises and programs that include eating certain types of food. To do this, you'll need to know your medical condition and what you can and cannot do.

If you have strong feelings of depression and worthlessness, even thoughts of suicide, I urge you to have a professional psychiatric or psychological evaluation.

♥ ♥ ♥

Now for the big question: CAN YOU CHANGE?

You may have read twenty diet books and another half dozen on behavior modification, and you may have tried every fashionable diet. But you haven't changed.

Can you change? Can you become different? Can you overcome your problems with food?

The answer: It depends.

IF you're looking for magic, the answer is no. *Magic* is my term to describe the people who try a highly restrictive diet, lose twenty-five pounds, and hold on to some magic belief that they will never regain the weight.

IF you're looking for an easy, comfortable, no-work-involved method that will make you thin, trim, and happy forever and ever, the answer is no.

IF you're willing to work at your problem—and it won't be easy—the answer is yes.

Change isn't easy. It's not comfortable. Making changes in your attitude or life-style (including your eating) can be a frightening and confusing experience.

So I want you to know before you read the next chapter, positive change demands work and commitment from you. You also need to know that whenever you make a positive change, many people around you will say, "I wonder if it's going to last." After all, they've watched you yo-yo for years. They may have heard you praise the newest diet or program, and then months later, you said, "It just didn't work."

I hope that knowing the difficulties that confront you, accepting the hard work you'll have to do, and facing the pessimism you'll have to overcome in yourself and your friends, you'll still decide to change.

I want to help you. I'll also show you how to get help. But most of all, I want you to commit yourself to facing your problem and winning the battle once and for all.

--------------------- ♥ ♥ ♥ ---------------------

Vital facts about myself: I acknowledge that I
have a problem with food, and I commit to
win over that problem.

--------------------- ♥ ♥ ♥ ---------------------

Can you change?

2

♥

My Real Problem Is...

I'm going to describe four people. See if you can figure out who has a food-related problem.

Melva. Melva's parents were obese. Even when she was a child, her parents and friends referred to her as big boned. She accepted that because she noticed she didn't eat any more than her friends, yet she seemed to be larger. When Melva was thirteen, she found it increasingly difficult to participate in gym class because of her weight. She was too embarrassed to go swimming. Melva described herself as feeling "fat" and "ugly." When she began college, she was fifty pounds over her ideal weight. Although she was certain she didn't eat more than her peers who were of ideal weight, she still gained three to five pounds a year.

Delbert. Delbert's family was dysfunctional. His father was an alcoholic. His mother had a controlling and perfectionistic personality; "Don't you ever do anything right?" was her favorite expression. During his teens, Delbert struggled with relationships because he didn't know how to interact with a girl. At age twenty, after a short romance and dating period, he married. A year later, Delbert began to be aware that every time his wife criticized him or asked him to do anything, he felt extremely hungry. He ate shortly after completing the task. He never gained much weight, but he felt out of control when criticized.

Craig. A high-energy sports enthusiast throughout his high-school career, Craig played baseball and was a hero to his

13

classmates and community. In his senior year of high school, he led his team to the state championship. He won a baseball scholarship to attend a college in his state. He made the team the first year, but he never played much. The second year his scholarship wasn't renewed, and he didn't make the baseball team. His identity had been taken away from him. He felt he was nobody; he was embarrassed and ashamed. Those feelings led him to munch on snacks whenever he was alone. He quit exercising and began putting on weight.

Eunice. She was brought up in a home where both parents were of normal weight, but she felt unloved by them. She enjoyed large breakfasts of bacon, eggs, and sausage every day. For lunch, Eunice ate sandwiches and chips and drank several glasses of soda. At dinner they always had meat, potatoes, two other vegetables, and dessert.

Eunice learned to enjoy food—lots of it. As she grew up, she became quite shy except around people she knew well. She ate large amounts of food at meals, snacked frequently, and insisted on desserts. She couldn't go to sleep without bedtime snacks.

Before Eunice was thirty years old, she was more than one hundred pounds over her ideal weight, even though she had gone on eleven different diets in five years.

Which one has the eating problem? Melva does. So does Delbert. Craig does, too. I'm sure you had no trouble deciding that Eunice fits into the problem category.

Now let's look at the types of food dependency problems in our society. These are problems of addiction. I have listed four types of addictions that can result in eating disorders. These are the major types of eating disorders I have encountered. You and each of the persons mentioned fit into one or more of these categories.

1. Genetic Addiction   *Melva*
2. Generational Addiction   *Delbert*
3. Situational Addiction   *Craig*
4. Compulsive Addiction   *Eunice*

1. GENETIC ADDICTION

Food dependency sometimes skips a generation, so your grandparents may have had a food problem. It's important to determine this information because many dependencies have a genetic component to them.

The genetic component of addiction can affect your weight loss program in three different ways. First, the genetic component may control your metabolism or general weight level. That is the most common form of genetic influence. It is similar to getting blue eyes or brown hair from your parents. Statistics indicate that if both your parents are overweight, one out of two children in your family will have a weight problem, even if they're not raised by their birth parents. If only one parent is overweight, the statistics suggest that one out of three children will have a food problem. I should note here that metabolism is also altered by quick weight loss/ starvation diets. Research is beginning to show that individuals who use quick weight loss programs tend not only to regain their initial weight but to gain additional weight as well.

Second, the genetic component may result in a predisposition to compulsive behaviors. There is some indication that people can inherit a "compulsive gene," which can cause any number of compulsive behaviors. In that way parents pass on to their children their dependency on chemicals (such as alcohol or drugs) and food.

Third, the genetic component may affect neurotransmission levels. That means that you could be "genetically depressed" or "genetically anxious," either of which could cause overeating.

2. GENERATIONAL ADDICTION

Generational addiction is passed on because of the way families *interact*. Genetic is biological; generational is learned or behavioral.

When compulsive overeating and other forms of addictive behavior are present in a family, we say, "They are a dysfunctional family." That is, an emotionally unhealthy family does not function by commonly accepted standards of its society.

If you grew up in a dysfunctional family, you were taught unhealthy ways to behave because of the way others in your family behaved. Long before you could ask if it was healthy, you absorbed some of these forms of conduct. I'll give you a few examples.

The screamer parent. Your father was a screamer. It was the one way to get what he wanted. Growing up, you unconsciously learned to raise your voice to its peak level. Like your dad, you got the attention. If you shouted loud enough, you got what you wanted.

The silent parent. Your mother was quiet, perhaps even silent, during stressful times. You had no idea how she felt because she never shared her emotions. Now that you are an adult, you may have realized that the more traumatic the situation, the quieter you become. You react that way because it is a learned pattern of behavior.

The nonangry family. Although no one may have actually said so, you learned that anger wasn't an acceptable emotion. Since it wasn't acceptable, you unconsciously learned to deny feelings of anger. Perhaps you also learned to swallow negative feelings.

All three of these characteristics of behavior (and many others) appear in dysfunctional families. The family system wasn't functioning right, and such behavior negatively affected you.

Generational addiction shows itself most frequently in the form of abuse. Because the term *abuse* is used so widely today, it may cause misunderstanding. I use the word *abuse* as an overarching term to include any of the following: harm, violate, assault, put down, mistreat, deprecate, diminish, belittle, condemn, hamper, block, denigrate, mishandle, misuse, damage, degrade, obstruct, or victimize.

I have identified several forms of generational abuse in dysfunctional families.

Spiritual abuse

Probably the most overlooked aspect of dysfunctional families (especially in the religious community) is that of spiritual abuse. Frequently in very religious families, parents have used their pious background to force their values on their kids. In essence they've said, "God wants you to behave this way, and if you don't, you'll be punished." Such demands are a form of spiritual abuse because they impose the parents' values instead of guiding and allowing the children to find their own.

Physical abuse

We know more today about physical abuse in dysfunctional families. You may have a problem with food because you were beaten, hit, or threatened, or you lived in fear of being hurt. This factor frequently occurs in generational addiction, especially with food dependencies.

Sexual abuse

Food addiction because of sexual abuse in childhood is extremely common. More than one expert in the field of sexual assault has said, "I have never seen a bulimic or an anorexic who did not have a history of sexual abuse." They are not saying that everyone who is a bulimic (someone who self-purges or vomits after eating) or an anorexic (someone who refuses to eat) is a victim of sexual assault, but there is a high statistical correlation between the two.

Sometimes it's difficult to pinpoint exactly, but sexual abuse essentially means violation of your body. Besides actually engaging in the sexual act, it includes caressing, hugging, and inappropriate touching. Any of these acts can contribute to the inner issues that trouble individuals later in life. (If sexual abuse has been part of your life, you will also deal with spiritual and emotional components that follow that form of abuse.)

Emotional abuse

Emotional abuse occurs when you're put down, criticized, made to feel unloved, or hindered from feeling your own feelings. You hear these comments:

- "You're not angry. You can't be angry over a little thing like that."
- "Stop that crying! You aren't hurt. If you don't stop, I'll really give you something to cry about!"
- "You've never done anything right in your life. What makes you think you'll ever change?"
- "I can't wait until you're out of high school. Then you're out of the house for good."
- "You don't have enough sense to know..."
- "You're a lazy, worthless good-for-nothing."

These statements are emotionally abusive because they are not loving and affirming. Many people grow up with such statements and accept them as true, regardless of the reality.

Intellectual abuse

Perhaps two illustrations can explain this abuse. First, I think of my friend David. Although he is extremely bright, he has never believed he was more than average in intelligence. David dismissed his high grades in college because of luck, because he studied hard, or because the professor graded easy.

David told me that when he was twelve years old, he and his family were standing together in a mall. His father pointed to a severely retarded boy and said to the rest of the family, "Hey, there goes David." Everyone else laughed. David turned his face away and shed silent tears.

Here is a second illustration. Anita's parents pushed her intellectually. They expected her to bring home perfect grades or at least the highest in her class. Whenever anyone else had as high a grade as Anita, her parents nagged her for not studying harder.

As she grew older, Anita internalized this fact: "I am loved and valued only if I perform intellectually and prove that I'm the best." Anita believed that if she fell short of being number one, she was a failure. The stress enabled her to graduate from high school and college at the top of her class. But Anita developed food-dependency issues and other psychological problems.

Victims of intellectual abuse heard these statements while growing up:

- "You're too dumb to go to college (or work in an office)."
- "If you were really smart, you would..."
- "Why do you bring in lousy grades? Why can't you be smart like...?"

Identity abuse

Some adults still don't know who they are. Perhaps they were middle children. Because they weren't the oldest or the youngest, they had no idea who they were.

Or they were just "different." "I didn't look like the rest of the family," cried Dawn. "They were all large boned and muscular. I was tiny, skinny, and frail looking."

You weren't good at sports and others were, so you were ignored. Other family members mixed well with people, but you were quiet, so you got neglected. Whatever the cause, you never developed a separate identity. Today, as an adult, you still haven't understood who you are.

3. SITUATIONAL ADDICTION

You turn to food because you are at that moment involved in a circumstance, situation, problem, or environment where food is a natural response to the pressures you're feeling. (This reaction is probably unconscious.)

Here are examples of such situations.

You had a tough day at the office. Immediately upon getting inside the house, you eat. The terrible, overpowering situation was the stress you felt at the office. Food was the drug you used to relieve the stress.

You're getting ready to go to work the next morning. As you think about your day, you anticipate the pressures. You pause to grab another doughnut and another cup of coffee. You feel a little better, a little more able to cope with what lies ahead of you.

You are the substitute teacher in your Sunday school class. Or you have to give a speech or a presentation for your company. The gnawing in your stomach may be nervous anxiety and fear, but you calm it by filling it with food.

If you use food in such situations often enough, you will train yourself to turn to food before or after every unpleasant circumstance. It won't be just when you face work-related stress. Before you go to the doctor or to a concert, you'll eat. Situational use means you *must* eat before or after or both times.

You'll probably say to yourself, "Hey, I was hungry. That's all. I just wanted to have a quick snack to tide me over..."

Because it's situational use of food, you probably won't want to admit it. You may well defend your behavior by saying something such as, "I don't overeat every day. I'm not one of those people who inhales food and has to eat all the time."

Situational use does not mean that you are so addicted that you have to keep your stomach stuffed with goodies every hour of the day. Situational use does mean that you use food under certain conditions and in particular settings. Because you turn to food during times of stress and discomfort, you have a food-dependency problem. Some of your friends turn to an antacid or aspirin. You eat away your upset stomach or headache.

By the way, if you're like most people, you probably fall into this category of situational addiction.

4. COMPULSIVE ADDICTION

Every time you start to eat, you can't stop until you are bloated and miserable. No matter how much willpower you exert, no matter how much you talk to yourself, you just can't push away from the table if there's anything left for you to ingest. You hate yourself for being that way, but you can't seem to stop. Food excites you, and eating takes precedence over everything else in your life. Even when you're not eating, food is on your mind; you're planning your next meals or reviewing your previous ones.

The good news is that only about 5 percent of persons with food-related problems fall into this category.

♥ ♥ ♥

Once you accept the type of food problem you have, you are already getting rid of another pitchfork load of unwanted muck.

Here is your self-affirmation:

♥ ♥ ♥

Vital fact about myself: I admit that my food-related problem falls into the categories of _____ and _____. I commit myself to change my attitude about food.

♥ ♥ ♥

3

— ♥ —

Your Life or Your Food

From movies and television, most of us know the old routine of a stranger coming up in a dark alley and snarling, "Your money or your life."

What happens when the voice says, "Your life or your food"? Which one is more important? Total honesty may make it hard for you to answer. You may respond,

- "Everybody has to eat. How can you ask me to make a choice? Why make a choice? Overeating is not the best for me, but it's not as if I get drunk all the time or snort cocaine."

- "I can stop eating whenever I want to. I just like food a lot. You think I'm addicted like some of those people who can't exist without a fix?"

- "Sure I'm overweight, and I struggle with my weight like most people do. But it's not something that makes me do weird things."

- "Oh, sure, eating is one of the few things I enjoy. Now I suppose I have to hear that it's some kind of uncontrollable addiction or that all food causes cancer or depletes the ozone layer. Give me a break. Just let me eat, okay?"

- "I have a weight problem, but I'm certainly not addicted to food. I don't eat more than anyone else. My metabolism is just different."

21

- "I am not addicted to food. Alcoholics can help themselves but don't, so they are addicted."
- "Me? I try to change, but I can't. It's part of my physical makeup. Addicts have a choice. I don't."

These are typical statements when words such as *food, life,* and *addiction* are linked together. No one wants to equate overeating or food-dependency problems with addiction. Unfortunately, many people deny their addiction to food. It's not socially acceptable to most of us to admit addiction to anything.

Some have argued that no one has an *addiction* to food itself. Literally, that's true. Food is only the substance you use to meet an unfulfilled need. If you have a food-dependent personality, you are lacking, deprived, or unsatisfied in some area of your life. You use food as a substitute for the real thing.

First, an illustration may clarify this point. Let's say it's Saturday evening, no one is around, and you feel lonely. (This is true even if you're not able to define or explain your emotion.) Because you feel a little on the lonely side, you eat two chocolate bars. By the time you have finished the candy, you are feeling less lonely. You have just substituted a *substance* to replace or fill an emotional need.

Further, part of the definition of addictive behavior is that it is a behavior you do automatically and often without conscious thought. You don't pause to consider your emotions or worry about the lack in your life to "do your drug." I would even say that you do it instinctively or habitually.

You ate the chocolate without thinking through why you were eating. It's not likely that before you took your first bite, you reasoned,

1. I feel lonely tonight. I feel as if nobody cares.
2. Eating will take the edge off my emotional need.
3. After I eat, I will feel less lonely.
4. I am going to eat now.

You were already feeling lonely, and before you defined the feeling for yourself, something inside your head whispered, "I'm hungry. I'd like a chocolate bar right now." So you ate.

Part of the nature of addiction is that it often hides or denies the source or cause of its cravings.

Suppose I came by to see you when you were still eating the candy, and I said, "You finished supper only twenty minutes ago. Why are you eating candy now?"

"I'm still hungry," you might say. "I just felt hungry for chocolate right now" might be another answer. You might even rationalize, "I decided before supper that I would eat the candy now." It's not that you would intentionally lie, but your defense system would come up with reasons and explanations.

You might come up with five seemingly valid reasons for eating the candy. Quite likely you have been giving yourself reasons for a long time, and now you don't even think about your need for more food. You just eat. You may wish that you didn't eat so much or that you could control the amount of food you put into your body. But you eat anyway.

One woman became quite upset at hearing me use *food* and *addiction* together. "I eat only when I worry," she said. "It calms my nerves." She continued, "I'm high-strung, and I know I worry too much." Doesn't that sound like situational addiction?

Unless it's a compulsive behavior that says you *must* eat and must eat *now* (the 5 percent I mentioned in the previous chapter), most people don't want to admit to food dependency. If you're like most people, you can stop eating in most situations. You probably can't avoid eating in those circumstances, but you can usually cut down the amount.

Don't be fooled into thinking an exercise of willpower means you are *not* food dependent. Dependency can exist even if you stop after reasonable servings. Dependency refers to the *effects* of food on your life. Whether you overeat once or twice a year or three or four times a week, it isn't how frequently you overeat, and it isn't how much you overeat. The question to ask yourself is this: Does eating interfere with my life?

When I used the word *interfere,* I immediately thought of Lila. She is an elfin ninety-eight pounds and stands just under five feet tall. No one would think that Lila has a food-dependency problem. But she does. Every day of her life, she agonizes over how much she can eat. Because she exerts an enormous amount of self-control, she eats the precious amount that keeps her weight below one hundred pounds. But she pays an enormous price for that lighter weight. Lila is under constant stress, feels edgy, and has started to smoke again after five years of abstinence.

Think about your life.

- Are the friends you socialize with constantly eating?
- Does food constitute your major form of relaxation?
- Do you plan your activities around eating?
- Do you feel bored if you have to go to a meeting where no food is served?
- Is food a primary topic of conversation?

If you answered yes, your social life is probably controlled by food. That indicates you have a problem.

Mentally examine your relationships. Do your spouse, kids, parents, grandparents, and others close to you tell you that you eat too much? Or that you're too concerned about food? If they do, food may be interfering in the relationships.

Reflect on your job or school attendance. I'm not referring to how often you go or whether you arrive on time. If you miss your coffee break or midmorning snack, do you feel a little bit slowed down? Are you sometimes aware that you're not quite at your best if you don't get a food pickup? That is a good clue for you to consider how food affects you vocationally.

Mull over your level of spirituality. Do you have trouble experiencing real peace? Is it difficult or impossible for you to define who you are? Do you wonder why you don't feel that you have a purpose in life? If you answer yes, food may be interfering with your spiritual life.

Consider your physical health. Is your health deteriorating? Have you realized that you're unable to do what you could do only a few years ago? Do you have a list of reasons why you're unable to exercise? If you answer yes, food may be interfering with your health.

If food interferes with the various areas of your life—social, relational, vocational/educational, spiritual, and physical—you have a problem.

When you're stressed out or anxious, do you grab a quick snack before you can start to relax? If something special and wonderful has happened and you want to celebrate, do you immediately think of food? If you find yourself looking to food first, food is interfering with your life.

An overuse of food doesn't mean you are incapacitated as if you had been drinking alcohol all night or had taken a handful of prescription drugs. But food is interfering with your life if you *need* it

- to get yourself in a good mood.
- to get ready to study or do your taxes.
- to fortify yourself before you go on a date or a job interview.
- to calm you down.
- to pick you up.
- to give you something to do with your hands so you won't be so nervous.

Food dependency interferes with life in other ways as well. Various psychological/personality, identification, and sociocultural issues are caused by and contribute to food-related problems.

PSYCHOLOGICAL/PERSONALITY ISSUES

Problems with food are caused by and lead to problems of the personality. These are what we call the psychological issues. As you read, ask yourself, Does this describe me?

Low self-esteem

How do you feel about yourself? Have you learned or accepted negative things about yourself? Do you think of yourself as inferior? Weak? Useless? Do you lack a strong feeling about just who you are?

Even if you feel confident in what you *do*, self-esteem may be an issue because you're not confident in who you *are*. Among persons with eating problems, a sense of low self-esteem is extremely common.

I'll say it more strongly: Of all the people I've worked with, everyone who has had a food-dependency problem has had low self-esteem.

Conditional love

Do you feel the way you are loved is based on how you perform or behave? If you do something terrible or mean, will the important people in your life still love you? If you fail or don't perform at a certain level, do they withhold love? Do their actions say, "I'll love you if..."?

Nonacceptance

Do you feel that you're never quite good enough? No matter how hard you work or try, you're sure that the important persons in your life won't accept you? Do you feel as if you are defective material? Do you think that if you changed and got better, you would feel more accepted?

You may believe that people around you—parents, spouse, and/or children—are asking you to be somebody that you aren't.

All of us make mistakes. But do you focus on your mistakes? Do you worry about where you messed up and what you *can't* do? Acceptance includes understanding that you make mistakes. You can't undo them, but you can learn from them. One of the things you can learn is that mistakes are not who you are.

Guilt

Do you have guilt feelings because of things you've done, even if they happened years ago? Or do you feel guilty, thinking, *I should have done more?* Do you feel responsible for everything that goes wrong at home or on the job? You may be thinking, *If I were who I should be, then...* No one would suffer or have problems if you did your duty. That's guilt. If you stop to examine those feelings, they are seldom logical, but they are often deep-seated.

Guilt may have been a device your parents used to manipulate you; you were so manipulated that even today you feel guilty for not being all-wise and all-powerful. If you feel guilty just for being human, you have a problem here.

Guilt is one thing that plagued Marie. Her parents lived through the Great Depression of the 1930s. When she was a child in the 1950s, they didn't allow her to leave any food on her plate. "When I was your age, I would have given anything to have that much food to eat in a whole day," her father said.

"If you only knew how we worried about having enough food and clothes just to get by," her mother often remarked, "you'd think three or four times before you would throw away the food on your plate."

Marie was a parent of teenagers before she realized that her parents used guilt as a means of control.

Shame and embarrassment

Shame refers to you as a person—who you are. Embarrassment refers to how you behave—what you do. It's bad enough to feel embarrassed when someone laughs at you for over-eating. It becomes a serious problem when you feel you are an unacceptable person because of your eating habits. That is shame.

Do you feel ashamed

- for being unable to control your appetite?
- for your lack of willpower?
- for being overweight?
- for being larger or bigger than other family members?
- for not being able to participate in activities with other family members?

Fear

Has fear been instilled in you? Fear shows itself in various ways:

- Fear of failing
- Fear of being physically abandoned (you're afraid that those you love will eventually leave you)
- Fear of emotional abandonment (those you love won't or don't love you; they may not actually leave, but they don't care about you)
- Fear of not being accepted by others
- Fear of not being respected

Performance

Do you feel that you just don't do a good enough job? No matter how hard you work or how long you slave over something, it's never quite perfect. Whether it's cooking or making furniture repairs or landscaping, the results are just not up to *their* level of expectation. (Sometimes you're not sure who your critics are.)

IDENTIFICATION ISSUES

The second area to consider is that of identification issues. Each of us has an identity, a *conception* of who we are. Usually that identity is based on a combination of characteristics that we hold in high esteem. Often, when we are young, our identity is based on our appearance and our abilities and is influenced by the opinions of our peers.

Physical attractiveness

Do you feel ugly? Unattractive? My friend Bob told me about an experience when he was in the army. He was so hairy, he felt as if a fur pelt covered his body. He was sure that the other men in his barracks would think of him as a wild man. He hated for the others to see him undressed.

One day he discovered that his best friend was just as inhibited for another reason. "I don't have a single hair on my chest," his friend said, "and I feel self-conscious about it. Sometimes I worry that others will think I'm not a real man because I can't grow any hair on my chest."

Bob said that both of them were finally able to laugh at themselves and realize that they had set up standards of how real men were supposed to look. "By those standards, neither one of us was attractive," he said.

Talent

Perhaps you have an outstanding talent. You're good enough so that you actively compete in sports, art, music, or another field. Yet, no matter how good you are, you still feel inferior. Or you really feel that you are less gifted than others.

You compare your achievements with those of your competitors. You're convinced that the others are better.

Or maybe it's the other way around. You have an outstanding talent that you accept and others recognize. Unfortunately, that talent becomes your identity. If you couldn't play the piano or football, you might not know your identity as a person.

Tom is one of the finest preachers I've ever listened to. He's so good, in fact, that church members, friends, and admirers kept urging him to publish. Tom decided to learn to write. One summer he attended a five-day writers' workshop.

"I was miserable the whole time," he said. "Nobody knew me or cared that I was a preacher. Writing was all they cared about. And for five days, I just didn't know who I was." I'm not sure that Tom understood why. His identity was so tied into being a preacher that when he wasn't recognized in that capacity, he didn't know who he was. Tom's talent had become his identity.

SOCIOCULTURAL ISSUES

The sociocultural element contributes to food dependency, and it revolves around how you were brought up. Do any of these issues pertain to you?

Poverty

Many persons brought up in real poverty felt deprived as children and continue to feel that way as adults. Food is one thing that makes them feel better. Because there was no money, they had little to do for relaxation. They might have used food for that purpose. As long as they have food—and plenty of it—they don't feel so impoverished.

Wealth

On the other hand, wealth can be equally a dynamic in creating food dependency. Because of your affluent background, it was appropriate for you to attend parties and outings regularly. You went to so many social occasions, you learned that interacting with others was always done around food.

Parental issues

Certain types of behavior that contribute to food dependency come from ways of doing things that you learned or imitated within your family.

Perfectionism. If your parents were perfectionists or demanded perfection from others, they might have temporarily eased their need to be perfect by turning to food. You may feel the only way to survive your imperfection is to use food to stuff your feelings inside.

Control. Do you often feel that you have to hold everything together? That you have to direct or tell others how to act or work? If a situation gets too tense, you quickly insert a joke or change the topic. You work at keeping the lid on so that everybody gets along. When situations are taken out of your control, do you feel angry? Stressed? Depressed? Does eating something alleviate your tension?

Workaholism. There is a difference between working hard and being controlled by your work. Workaholism is compulsive activity. You *have* to work; you can't leave your job behind; you think about it constantly.

Maybe you grew up in a workaholic family. Children whose parents are pastors, doctors, teachers, and social workers often complain that their parents' work came first. They didn't feel loved. Or if they did, the work of their parents was more loved.

If you had workaholic parents, perhaps you were made to feel that you were not as important as your parents' ministry, profession, or occupation. If you felt unloved or rejected, turning to food would be an obvious way to cope with the situation.

If you are the workaholic, you experience tremendous stress. A voice says within you, "I have to keep working. I need to do more. I have to accomplish more." You bury yourself in productivity instead of developing wholesome relationships. Then you turn to food for consolation over your plight.

Compulsive overeating. If one of your parents was a compulsive overeater, you have a higher statistical chance of using food to take care of your emotions. Some compulsive overeaters stop their habit and replace food dependency with alcohol or drugs. Or perhaps you were addicted to drugs or alcohol but now use food instead. If you have done that, we say that you have *transferred* your addiction. You have not resolved your issues, only hidden them in a different place.

♥ ♥ ♥

The issues involved are complex. The causative factors can be any of these or a combination from genetic to generational to psychological to physical to sociocultural issues to compulsive behavior in the background.

In the last two chapters, I've been trying to push you to focus on these factors. I want you to be able to identify them. Then you can say, "That's where it came from, and these are the effects it's having on my life." That will then lead you to the obvious questions: Now where am I going to go? What do I do about it?

♥ ♥ ♥

Vital facts about myself: I am a valuable, worthwhile human being. I have a problem with food. I am not the problem.

♥ ♥ ♥

4

♥

Your Food or Your Health

In the last chapter, I asked you to consider an important question: Does eating interfere with my life? Now I want you to ponder a more specific question: Does eating interfere with my health?

If you are food dependent, regardless of the amount you eat, this problem affects you physically. And if it affects you physically, it also has an effect on your emotions.

First, I want to look at your physical health. Then I'll look at how it affects your emotional health.

FOOD AND PHYSICAL HEALTH

When I speak of the effects of improper eating on your physical health, even if you haven't felt the effects of poor health, you are setting up your body for pain and sickness.

If you rigidly control your amount of food, you may be a purger. A number of serious physical effects result from regular purging or self-induced vomiting, such as absorption problems, potassium deficiency, heart irregularities, stomach ulcers, weakness of the muscles, and improper nerve function.

If you strictly monitor the amount of food you eat, the chances are that you will choose food on the basis of caloric value and not that of nutrition. You will suffer from not getting the nutrients your body needs. Any number of diseases, such as hypertension, arteriosclerosis, and osteoporosis, may be direct results of an improper food balance.

Too much food almost acts like poison to your body because it will destroy your health or create disease within your body. Conditions such as high cholesterol levels and diabetes are severe problems in themselves, and they can cause you to lose immunity to other diseases, shorten your life, and affect your attitude.

When you stop medicating yourself with food, eat sensibly, and change your life-style, you can reverse many of these conditions. If you are among the majority of individuals, when you make these changes early enough, they probably won't have shortened your life or your quality of life. If you have abused your body so that your health is already seriously affected, you can still improve your health and probably enjoy life much more.

FOOD AND EMOTIONAL HEALTH

Now, let's look at food and your emotional health. Here is your self-affirmation:

♥ ♥ ♥

Vital fact about myself: What I eat affects my health and my emotions. Because I want to be physically and emotionally well, I am learning about and changing my eating habits.

♥ ♥ ♥

The truth—and maybe this seems too obvious—is that you can overcome any problem you can admit to having. One reason your obstacles remain unresolved is that you don't face them.

Suppose your foot hurts so much you limp and feel a shooting pain every time you put your weight on it. I observe this, and I ask, "What's wrong with your foot?"

"Oh, nothing, really."

"But you're limping. You wince in pain," I insist.

"No big deal," you say. "Just hurts when I walk."

I respond, "Let me look at it. I think I know how to take away your pain. You'll never have to limp again."

If I then tell you three simple things to do for a complete cure, what would you do? You'd do the three simple things, wouldn't you? You'd say, "I'm so tired of this pain, I'm willing to do anything."

I'm saying the same thing about your problem with food. This book can tell you what to do and how to do it. If you will follow the steps outlined in this book, you can be functional once again.

I've observed that people with food-dependency issues have the following common emotional problems. These problems often interfere with recovery.

Denial

This problem is the most frequent and troublesome. Food dependency isn't like addiction to cigarettes or drugs. The tendency, even among persons who have gone this far into a program, is still to say in their hearts, "Oh, I don't eat the way I should. I just haven't paid much attention to eating properly. It's just a matter of deciding to eat right and doing it." That's denial.

Or some people compare themselves to a friend or coworker: "Look at Linda. She must weigh three hundred pounds. I'm not in any kind of shape like that."

Others say, "I can lose weight anytime I want to. I do it all the time. Just a little more effort and it's done." Such individuals don't accept the reality that they regain the weight. If they don't regain the weight, they still have a problem as long as they continue to suffer by battling over food.

Even some persons of normal weight are not free from food dependency. They devote so much of their energy and thinking to food and weight control, they are never at peace. If this stress remains long enough, it affects them physically.

These are all ways of denying the underlying problems.

A few people deny their food dependency because they have been programmed to think that if they are overweight, they are lazy and useless.

"My dad always said that if you want anything done," admitted Don, "you never ask a fat person to do it. They're all lazy." As he spoke to me, he looked at his expanded form and said, "I don't want to think of myself as no good."

I want you to know that you can change. No matter how

deep-seated your problem with weight, you are not of less value than anyone else.

Anger

The second most common problem centers on anger. Right now you're probably experiencing anger. You are angry that you have a food-dependency issue or that you're obese. You may have stored up anger against all sorts of things in life because life really isn't fair.

Anger comes in many forms. Maybe you call it resentment, hostility, or frustration. Sometimes it's an out-of-control rage. Among many Christians, anger is considered unacceptable, so they tend to deny its existence. They think that if they're angry, they can't be good Christians—maybe not even real Christians.

Anger is normal for everyone. You may have an inordinate amount because you can't or won't bring your anger to the surface. But anger is part of the dependency issue.

If you have difficulty acknowledging anger, use this self-affirmation:

♥ ♥ ♥

Vital facts about myself: I accept my anger. It is all right to feel my anger. I separate my anger from my eating habits.

♥ ♥ ♥

Blaming

You may blame your parents, your spouse, your family, or your body for your problems—all can contribute to food dependency. But blaming won't help. Understanding your views of stress and stressful situations can help you stop blaming others. Knowing that genetics or metabolism may contribute to your food dependency is important, but you are the one who must live in this situation or change.

Withdrawal

Often persons with food-dependency problems change their life-style and begin to withdraw. Perhaps you feel unattractive, so you avoid being with the public. Perhaps you avoid social events that involve physical activity or exercise because you feel inadequate.

Distorted thinking

A factor that can interfere with your recovery is distorted thinking. Distorted thinking shows up when you believe that

- you can't change.
- your efforts are useless.
- your metabolism and genetics keep you in this cycle.
- you aren't liked by others because of your food dependency.

To this point, you have learned about the ways in which food dependency interferes with your life and, specifically, with your physical and emotional health. Now it is time to begin planning a recovery program that will change all that. The first thing you need is support.

5

— ♥ —

Essential Support

"It's wonderful!" Marcie said. For five months, she had followed a sound diet program and lost more than forty pounds. Next she started to change her life-style and learn healthy eating habits.

Sixty-nine days later, Marcie went on a compulsive binge. "I ate everything in the kitchen that didn't move," she whimpered. "And it wasn't just that night. I've been going like this for five days." She had already regained eight pounds.

"What kind of support system do you have?" I asked. "And has it helped?"

Marcie stared at me as if I had spoken in a foreign language. "Support system?" she echoed. "I don't know what you mean."

Marcie had other issues involved, but for her, the crucial need was a support system. She was not alone. If you want to recover from your eating problems, you can do it on your own. You may even be successful. But if you do it alone, you probably stand with about 1 percent of the American population. In fact, if you can do it all on your own, you probably don't need this book. BUT if you're like thousands of others I've worked with, and if you want to recover fully from food dependency, you need a support system.

You help yourself in your recovery, and you also learn to trust others more and to receive help and guidance from them—things you may not be good at receiving. And people who support you are rewarded by being able to help someone else.

God created all of us to interact. This is one way you can do that.

Most people need a support *system* and a support *person*. The system is a group or a fellowship to whom you are accountable. Your support person is the individual you contact between group meetings. In Overeaters Anonymous, the support person is known as a sponsor.

Please accept this truth: A support system is *not* an option. You need help from others to recover.

Because personalities differ, some may feel comfortable with a support person but not a group. Others may find groups helpful but be intimidated in a one-to-one situation. You will have to decide what you can do. Using both is ideal, but at least seek out a group *or* a person.

♥ ♥ ♥

I'm going to answer the most common questions and objections I receive about a support system for persons recovering from food dependency.

"ISN'T IT BETTER TO GO SOMEPLACE LIKE A RESIDENCE CLINIC?"

Some persons with addictive problems go away for treatment to clinics, rehab centers, and hospitals. Many of them find the help they need. The advantage, of course, is that in a hospital-type environment, you can escape the daily pressures that have been mounting up. You may need a vacation from stress. If you stay in your home environment, you may become dysfunctional.

Checking into a hospital may get you away from a pressurized environment, but you don't get away from yourself and your needs. It's difficult to stay among family, friends, and daily situations and make changes. However, in the long run, it may prove easier. At some point, you will have to return to your environment and learn to cope without using food as a medication or stimulator.

Because of the high level of success I've had with persons just like you, I want you to know that you can get help while living at home. By reading and using this material, you can become victorious over your food dependency. But you must deal with the issues on the battlefield. That way, you are not setting up artificial situations.

"I went to clinic after clinic," said one woman. "I got a lot of help. But when I got home and faced my family and job pressures, I knew it was only a matter of time before I went back to the clinic. With all the help and support I got there, I didn't know how to face the day-to-day problems here."

"WHAT CAN A SUPPORT SYSTEM DO FOR ME?"

Here are nine basic things that your support system can do for you.

1. Your support system helps you share your feelings

You will learn to share—but only as much as you can. Just by opening yourself to others, you experience hope. You discover that your problems are not as unique as you thought.

In a sharing group, my friend Hank said, "It's amazing to me, but when I really open up to my group and share the things that are the hardest to talk about, I learn that they understand. Instead of rejecting me, they embrace me. They say things like, 'I've felt that way myself.' It's so freeing."

You learn to share your problems and expectations. Others can feel your pain, understand your problems, and care about your welfare.

Deanne said, "I grew up in a family where I was called special. I was the star, the one who accomplished things. I compensated with a lifetime struggle with food. But one day in a support group, someone said to me, 'You know, Deanne, you are talented, but you're also quite ordinary.'"

Tears filled Deanne's eyes as she said, "That was when I knew how much I needed people to support me. They didn't elevate me to some pedestal, but they made me feel ordinary, just like the rest of them."

2. Your support system encourages you

One reason for having a support system is that you'll get discouraged at times. You'll be too hard on yourself and not want to forgive yourself for failing or not making faster progress. You'll tend to focus on what you have *not* accomplished instead of looking at how far you have come.

People in your support system can listen to you say,

- "I just want to give up."
- "I'm tired of fighting."
- "Is it worth it?"
- "I don't know if I want to do this anymore."

Your support person will be able to say, "You have come so far. You've fought a good fight, and you're going to win. I've watched you struggle, and I know you can make it."

Your support system

- renews your hope.
- points to your success, even though it's not complete.
- enables you to recognize that you may have had a setback in your recovery, but you haven't failed.
- challenges you to keep on.
- assures you that you can win your private war against food dependency.

A good support system will motivate you, stand loyally behind you, and encourage you when you're down. A support system is your personal cheerleading squad.

3. Your support system provides your reality check

No matter how much you try to focus inwardly, you can't see yourself objectively—no one can. You need individuals you can trust to view you objectively and still accept you. Your support system can help you learn to accept the things about yourself that you may not want to know but need to know. This is a *reality check*.

Particularly in the first weeks of recovery from food dependency, you need somebody to help you determine if what you think you see and understand is really what is going on.

During that transition time, you are most apt to misperceive reality.

As you work with your support system, ask questions such as:

- "Does this make sense?"
- "Here's what I was thinking, but it seems weird..."
- "Please tell me if I'm understanding this correctly."

That's reality checking. You have been a person with a food-related problem. Your overeating has affected your perceptions. You don't—you can't—always see yourself the way others do. That's one of the realities of your food-related addiction. You need someone who is honest and will tell you when your thinking is veering away from reality.

4. Your support system assists you in setting your priorities

You can do this yourself, but you probably need outside help.

Catherine wrote a list of priorities and took it to her group. "What are you going to do about your anger?" asked one member of the group.

"Why, I seldom get angry," she said. "That's not one of my issues—"

"Yes, it is," the person insisted. "It comes out with a type of teasing that you do—a lot—but it's not nice teasing. It's loaded with hostility. You smile when you talk that way, so it's not supposed to be interpreted as anger. But it is."

All five members of the support group had recognized Catherine's anger as one of her high-priority issues. She had been unaware of her own hostility.

5. Your support system calls you to accountability

You need to be accountable to somebody. You can think about your problems and make decisions. You may even write out a list and tape it on your bathroom mirror or on the refrigerator. Later, when you don't do what you promised yourself, you find ways to rationalize your lack of results. Or else you eat out of more guilt.

Instead, decide on your immediate goals. Tell your support person. Perhaps you set an unrealistic goal for yourself, and you are setting yourself up to fail. Or you set a reasonable goal, but you don't follow through. Your support person will ask, "Why didn't you do it?"

By using this book, you are actually going through a program that will show you what you need to do. Your supporter helps you decide if you are being responsible.

6. Your support system assists you in self-identification

You may find somebody else who is also recovering from food dependency. That person says, "You know, I went through that. I know exactly the stage you are in. Let me tell you what I did." It helps to know that somebody else has been down the road ahead of you, has made it to the end, and is willing to give you a hand. This person helps you identify where you are on the journey and accept that you are an all-right person.

7. Your support system guides you in bonding with others

You learn to lean on and to open up to somebody who is not going to hurt you. You learn how to begin and develop healthy relationships. One problem of food dependency is the fear of trusting or simply the inability to trust.

"I wanted to be understood," Ellen said, "but I had been laughed at as a child when I tried to express how I felt. I was afraid to let anyone else know how I felt. Then in desperation over my weight, I joined a support group. They knew what I was going through. They understood. Now I feel as if I am part of the group. I belong."

8. Your support system aids in your growth

Instead of focusing constantly on your weaknesses, a support system provides the challenge to look forward, to measure growth, to celebrate achievement. A support person and group focus on what you *are* and not on your failures or what you used to be.

For instance, I don't believe in saying, "My name is John. I am an overeater." John may need to say that in Stage 1 of his recovery, but as he moves on to Stage 2, he is striving toward living a balanced life. (Later, I explain the stages of recovery.) Everyone is not something—not musically inclined, not brilliant, not athletic—but the emphasis needs to be on who you are now and who you are becoming. Otherwise, you'll continue to feel inadequate. If you are involved with a healthy support group, you are growing. You share your growth and development with them.

9. Your support system helps you hear the truth in love

A support person should speak the truth in love. You need someone who can speak truthfully and faithfully in a spirit that also says, "I love you." That is different from brutal honesty that takes no account of human emotions. You need honesty. It will help if you say to your prospective support person, "You may get upset with me, but please tell me the truth anyway. I'm depending on you to help me."

"HOW DO I SELECT A SUPPORT PERSON?"

1. You can select your support person through a mutual help group such as Overeaters Anonymous

You can get that through what is called sponsorship—somebody who has been in recovery for a period of time and is willing to take you on personally.

As you consider that sponsor person and that sponsorship, I encourage you to go to a few meetings, look around, and choose somebody you can respect and interact with. Your support person is somebody you want to be honest with you, somebody who doesn't seek your approval and is willing to share right up front.

2. You can select a family member

Getting someone within your family involved can be extremely helpful—if the person can function with honesty and love. You don't need a family member who will criticize or belittle you. You don't need a family member who helps you set up a complaint session, either.

3. You can select a friend

If you choose your best friend, there may be hidden agendas. The friendship may be so valuable (or fragile) that the friend can't be as honest as you need that person to be. It may also be difficult for you to be fully honest with your friend.

4. You can select a minister or pastor

Not all ministers understand the issues of food dependency. But most counseling ministers and pastors understand what it means to provide support. As you read this book, you receive information about how to change and what is going on. A minister can support you as you learn.

"WHAT KIND OF SUPPORT GROUPS ARE AVAILABLE?"

There are two distinctive types of support systems available to you while you live at home.

Fellowship and twelve-step groups such as Overeaters Anonymous

These mutual help fellowships have been around for years. They have been quite effective. Visit such a fellowship. Attend a few sessions and see if it meets your needs. If you're not comfortable with a particular group of OA, most cities have several such groups that meet weekly. Each group has a different personality. If you are still uncomfortable, try another option.

Religious groups

Unfortunately, some church and religious groups may be the last place you want to go for support. You feel they all think that if you overeat, it's a sin and you're going to be punished. All churchgoers are not like that. Ask your pastor about a support group, or get help to know how to set up one.

A small group within the congregation. You may be active in a church and participate in Sunday school or the choir or a women's missionary group. Any of them could function as a support group.

Prayer groups. A prayer group is one of the most powerful places to learn how to communicate and share your feelings.

Bible studies. There are numerous Bible studies, men's groups, and women's groups. They can be immensely helpful.

"HOW DO I KNOW WHICH IS THE BEST SUPPORT GROUP?"

There is no "best" type. The best for you is based on your personality. Here's an example. A physician came to see me when I first started to work with compulsive behavior.

"Doc, I've got a problem," he said. "I think I'm an alcoholic. The laboratory profile I ran says I have a problem."

I was confused because he wasn't denying or hiding his addiction. I said to him, "Okay. What does your spouse think?"

"She doesn't think I have a problem."

"What do your office staff think?"

"They don't think I have a problem."

"And your kids?" I asked. "What do they think?"

"The same. They don't think I have a problem."

Then I was really confused. He was sure he had a problem, but no one else was. I wasn't sure how to counsel him. So I said, "I'd like you to go to a support group—Alcoholics Anonymous." (That was my method in those early days—referral first to AA.)

He went to an AA group meeting. When he came to see me again, he said, "I didn't like it, and I don't like AA."

"That's a problem," I said, citing my textbook knowledge. "Obviously, you have pride at stake, and your ego is holding you back." To his credit, the physician listened, even though he didn't like my words. Finally, I said, "Look, try again. Go to a different AA group."

He did exactly what I asked, but he still didn't like AA. I said, "You've got to get into the fellowship. You've got to get involved."

"If that's all you're going to tell me, I don't want to see you anymore," he replied.

I realized that he was serious. So I called Bob, a friend who had been in recovery and had attended AA for twelve years. I asked him if he'd have breakfast the next morning with the physician. He gladly accepted.

The following week, I asked the physician, "How did your breakfast go?"

"Which breakfast?"

"Hey, come on. The breakfast with Bob, my friend."

He laughed. "Yeah, but which breakfast with Bob? I went to breakfast with Bob three times. You know, Joel, I love the AA principles."

Then it hit me. The physician didn't like the way it was delivered in the groups, but he loved the concept. Because he was uncomfortable in the group situation, he couldn't "hear" the principles.

Who you are will determine how you respond and to whom you respond. You may not be comfortable in groups. That's all right. Connect instead with a support person.

"WHAT DO I ASK FOR WHEN I WANT SUPPORT?"

You need four things.

1. Ask about telephone privileges. (If you infringe on your support person's family system or privacy, the person will pull back from you.)

Ask specific questions, such as:

   • "When are you available by phone?"
   • "Can I call you anytime?"
   • "Is the middle of the night all right?"
   • "What about after supper?"
   • "Are you available during the daytime?"

2. Ask about showing your journal. You will probably want to keep a journal, daily if possible. In your journal record your feelings and attitudes, especially what you think and feel about food and eating.

When you meet with your support person, you may want to ask,

- "Is it all right if I show you part of my journal?"
- "You will keep this information confidential, won't you?"
- "Will you give me honest responses to what I write?"

If you ask these questions, they also imply that you will be open and willing to listen to your support person's responses.

3. Ask about visits:

- "When can we get together?"
- "Can we set up a routine time? Maybe breakfast every Tuesday and Thursday, or dinner on Monday and Thursday?"
- "If keeping the appointment presents any difficulty, will you let me know? I promise to do the same."

4. Ask about crisis availability:

- "If I'm in a crisis, will you be available?"
- "What do you consider a crisis?"
- "Will you help me distinguish between a problem and a crisis?"

Some people live from one crisis to another and seldom have days go by without one or two catastrophes. If you are such a person, I urge you to use group support. If you use only a support person, that person will burn out quickly. One of the worst things for you is to bond with your support person, only to be told, "I can't do this anymore. I'm getting depressed and burned out."

"WHAT SHOULD I NOT EXPECT OF MY SUPPORT PERSON?"

Your support person isn't your mother, father, God, best friend, or an infallible person. Here are three things to remember so that you don't ask, demand, or expect more than most support persons can deliver.

1. Your support person will be unavailable at times

You may be in a crisis, so you call. The person can't make you the center of life and be available every time. If you know that in advance, you won't get frustrated and depressed.

Suppose your support person says, "I'm sorry, but I'm not available to talk now."

You then ask, "When is a good time?"

2. Your support person will have other commitments

Don't take the unavailability as rejection. It is a way of saying, "I have other things going on in my life. I can't help you right now."

You are not the only thing in that support person's life. The person agreed to be your support and is willing to help as much as possible.

3. Your support person will get frustrated with you

That's common. At some point, everybody gets frustrated with the process. You may promise to do something. Yet when you meet the next time, you haven't fulfilled your commitment. If you do this several times, your support person will feel frustrated with you.

Your support person cares about you and wouldn't be working with you if he or she didn't care. It is precisely because your supporter cares and desires your growth that frustration happens. Instead of taking frustration as a form of rejection, say to yourself, "I disappointed my supporter. The person really does care about me."

♥ ♥ ♥

Vital facts about myself: I need a support system to help me with my food problem. I commit myself to setting up a support system to help me with my food-dependency problem.

♥ ♥ ♥

TIPS FOR THOSE WHO WANT TO BE PART OF A SUPPORT SYSTEM

Supporting persons who are recovering from addictions is a difficult task. The responsibility of properly supporting persons is an essential factor if they are to fully recover.

The following guidelines can help you decide whether you want to be involved in the support system. Not being part of the support system doesn't mean you are uncaring. If you sincerely feel you lack the needed qualities, say so. This process involves the life of another human being.

But don't be scared away, either. If you are willing to try to give your best, you may be just what that already hurting person needs.

I'd like you to visualize yourself standing before a person in recovery. Below are twelve statements. The first four have to do with WHO YOU ARE; numbers five through twelve revolve around WHAT YOU DO.

Try to see yourself facing that person. Imagine yourself raising your right hand and pledging your commitment.

1. "I am a stable, healthy person, and I want to help"

Not perfect, not fully accomplished, but you know who you are. You're balanced, you're together, and you like who you are, even though you're still putting the finishing touches on your life.

If you're balanced and healthy, you

- encourage instead of berate and condemn.
- offer options instead of saying, "This is the *only* way."
- allow others to grow at their own pace.
- understand when they fail because you remember your own failures.
- feel their struggles because you have struggled.
- trust because you have learned to trust God and others.

2. "I know my own limitations"

Often the best support comes when persons in recovery admit that they need something more than you can provide. You may suggest

- talking to a minister.
- consulting someone from their own cultural, ethnic, or racial background.
- seeking professional help, such as a therapist or physician.

When you feel uncomfortable and beyond your depth, be ready to suggest options for them to handle their particular issue.

3. "I am organized and ready"

An effective support person schedules routine times to talk with those in recovery. You discuss

- what they accomplished.
- what they didn't do.
- why they didn't complete what they agreed to.
- ways to make changes.

You may also suggest that they start keeping a journal. Each day they can write down their goals and objectives for that day.

4. "I am not a professional counselor"

The role of a support person is to provide encouragement, accountability, acceptance, reality checks, and opinions. Limit your "counseling" to being physically and emotionally present and suggesting options. To grow, persons in recovery need to make their own mistakes and achieve their own successes. You don't make decisions for them, but you support *them* when they make choices—even if you think they are unwise choices.

5. "I accept you without conditions"

Many people appear kind, loving, and considerate, but they struggle with feeling accepted. The greatest gift you can offer anyone is unqualified acceptance.

Acceptance means you allow persons to grow by looking at the process more than at their accomplishments. Their achievements or changing behavior can be slow, much slower than their understanding and insight.

6. "I accept and reinforce your accountability"

Accountability is one of the main roles of the support person. That includes asking what the person's goals are, challenging the person to work on the goals, and encouraging the person for achieving goals. If the person changes a goal, you can help determine whether the person is quitting or avoiding or has discovered a better option.

7. "I do whatever I can to build you up"

Making mistakes can be a learning experience, especially if you give support and encourage the person to get up, brush off, and move on. Criticism is rarely accepted as constructive. Encouraging and focusing on the positive are better ways to motivate change.

8. "I will listen—really listen—when you speak"

An effective support person doesn't offer suggestions or come to conclusions without hearing every side of the discussion. Your role isn't to decide who is right—after all, you're not asked to be a judge—but to help those in recovery understand their thoughts and feelings. When they speak, they may not "hear" what they are saying about themselves. If you listen with your full attention, you may be able to point out things they don't realize they said until you repeat the words. You can help by presenting other viewpoints and suggesting options. You can train yourself to listen to all the information and not get caught up in the crisis.

Remember, your concern isn't to figure out right or wrong or who's guilty. Your role is to understand.

9. "I learn, and I keep on learning"

You'll never know everything about supporting others, but you can learn much from experience and from caring.

To be effective as a support person, you need to learn as

much as you can about addiction. That includes neurochemistry, rewards, compulsive behavior, and the importance of following plans for diet, activity, and behavior. It's easier to encourage when you know the plans and the reasons behind the plans.

10. "I help you set priorities and goals"

Persons in recovery may need to be slowed down. Or they may need to be gently nudged. Some individuals in recovery want to attack all their problems at once. Others focus on an unchangeable issue of life, such as a medical problem or a disability. When people have something that can't be changed ever or at that time, support persons can encourage them to accept those things. Understanding when to motivate and in what areas is crucial.

11. "I am aware of your need for intimacy"

You also imply, "I know the difference between your need for intimacy, your tendency toward romantic attractions, and your pull toward sexual activity."

Whether you're married or single, if the recovering person is of the opposite sex, refuse to be the primary support person.

Intimacy and sexuality are difficult for many to separate. A certain bond develops when you help and care deeply for another. If you feel the pull to be more than a support person or are getting angry with the response of the recovering person's spouse, do both of them a favor and become a friend, not a support person.

12. "I provide reality checks"

Persons in recovery really do need reality checks. If you can question their "reality" in a supportive fashion and get them to explain how they came to such a conclusion, you are well on the way to providing the reality check they need.

♥ ♥ ♥

Can you be part of a support system?

To be asked means the recovering person has confidence in

you. Consider this responsibility seriously. But also consider it joyfully.

Jesus said it like this: "Whenever you did this for one of the least important of these brothers [or sisters] of mine, you did it for me!" (Matt. 25:40 TEV).

6

— ♥ —

The Fat in Your Head

Norman had just finished a thoroughly satisfying meal with his family. "I couldn't eat another bite," he told his wife. Actually, he felt a little stuffed so he decided to walk through a nearby mall.

He started to pass Baskin-Robbins. "The next thing I knew, I came out licking a triple-decker cone," Norman moaned. "And I wasn't even hungry. Am I crazy or something?"

"Not crazy, Norman, but something. That 'something' is in your head. It often has little to do with your stomach or hunger. You didn't eat again because you were hungry. You ate for other reasons. Think back, Norman. What was going on with you before you bought the ice cream?"

"Hmmm," Norman considered. "I was thinking about my job. We've heard from corporate headquarters that eight hundred employees will be cut this year. The rumor mill is saying that two hundred will come from our plant."

"How does this affect you, Norman?"

"I may be one of the two hundred out of a job in two months," he said.

"Norman, do you begin to understand why you ate when you weren't hungry?"

This chapter is about people like Norman. It's about you, your brain, and your brain chemistry (or your neurochemistry). You may be tempted to skip all or part of this chapter. Don't. This information is essential to your recovery.

THE IMPORTANCE OF NEUROCHEMISTRY

You need to know several things about the chemicals in your brain:

- They create your thoughts.
- They change your thoughts.
- They determine whether you perceive realistically.
- They cause you to seek rewards. (Rewards are the good feelings or the lessening of bad ones.)
- They stimulate your *reward center*. (I use this term to refer to the part of the brain that causes you to feel good or lessens a negative feeling when it is stimulated.)

Here is the most significant principle involved in making permanent changes, whether it refers to diet, behavior, or thinking:

♥ ♥ ♥

No one makes permanent changes
unless they pay off in a reward of
some kind.

♥ ♥ ♥

Consider these examples:

- As an average student, you study hard and get the best grade in class on a test. You get rewarded by the grade, the recognition, and the feeling of satisfaction with your efforts.
- As a child, you were told to pick up your toys or you would be spanked. You picked up the toys out of fear of being punished if you refused. Your reward came from *not* being punished.
- You have a job. Every two weeks you get a check.

Your money is your reward, even if you don't like
your job or your coworkers. You can pay your bills
and buy items you want.

I want you to learn about your brain chemistry. Later in this
book, I'm going to ask you to complete some questions for a
neurochemical evaluation. In fact, you must do your neurochemical evaluation to determine what you need in the way of
activity therapy, a sensible eating plan, and behavioral
changes. Above all, the combination of activity, food choices,
and behavioral changes needs to result in a reward.

For one thing, as you go through your diet recovery, you will
need a form of exercise. But which kind of exercise will give
you the biggest reward? Is running every day good for you?
What about low-impact aerobics? You probably don't know. If
you are like most people, you will tend to choose an exercise
that encourages your present form of behavior. If you are
already swimming or pumping iron, this form of exercise may
not be the best form of exercise for you.

In another chapter you will read about food choices. The
question is not, Which foods do you like? It is, Which foods do
you need? Most people in diet recovery have no idea how to
make intelligent food choices. They can follow diet plans. They
are experts, and why not? They've done that for years. They
can quote caloric or fat content, but they know little about
what they personally need to eat to reward themselves and to
alter their moods.

At this point, I want to add a word of caution. If you are food
dependent, you have a chemical imbalance *right now.* You can
change that, and I'll show you how. But your tendency will be
to avoid change. More than likely, you will want to transfer
your addiction. That is, you will stop overeating or misusing
food. But you won't balance the chemicals in your brain because you will do something else that involves exactly the
same chemical imbalance. You may take up smoking, become
a perfectionist, or get caught up in romance addiction. Some
people begin as alcoholics. When they stop drinking, they turn
to food dependency. They switch the form of the addiction, but
they don't free themselves of the problem or change their
themes.

AN EXPLANATION OF
NEUROCHEMISTRY

There are several elements to examine when defining neurochemistry.

First, neurochemistry refers to your nervous system and how the nerves in your brain interact. Your brain is filled with thousands of nerves that are similar to electrical wires. As you probably know, an electrical wire carries electricity in the form of impulses. Your brain works the same way.

Second, your sensory input—such as sight, touch, smell, and taste—brings in information through the nervous system. When this information reaches your brain, you have to interpret what you saw, touched, smelled, or tasted. You interpret that in your brain through individual nerves.

Third, what happens if you develop a break in your electrical wiring? Can you still carry electricity? Absolutely not. Your brain is equipped from birth with synapses or breaks in the nerves. These synapses act as dimmer switches so that they can modulate or monitor whether you are going to run fast, slow down, stay awake, or fall asleep. A synapse selectively releases chemicals in the break to cause the nerve to transmit information faster or slower. You can change or observe the extent of the reaction to the sensory input through your response by using your muscles to run faster, slow down, or relax.

Let's go back to the broken wire. The only way you can get electricity past the gap is for it to jump across the empty space. Your brain does that by releasing chemicals. These chemicals start from one side that has electricity. They jump across the chasm to the other side where they connect with nerves. This action makes the electricity continue. It creates the movement or even the feeling that occurs on the other end. These chemicals are then broken down by enzymes. The faster the enzyme, the shorter the action of the chemical.

Fourth, at any given time, you have in your brain what I call gas-pedal chemicals and brake-pedal chemicals. These neurochemicals are transmitted from one side of the nerve to the other. Since you have both a gas pedal and a brake pedal, you have two choices to speed you up. You can (*a*) push down on the gas pedal or (b) pull back on (or release) the brake pedal. If you want to slow down, you again have two choices. You can (a) push down on the brake pedal or (b) pull back on the gas pedal.

The amounts of gas-pedal chemicals and brake-pedal chemicals vary in your brain according to what you are doing. They won't be the same when you are running from fear as they are when you are running for pleasure. When you are anxious, they differ from the moments when you are depressed.

Fifth, I stress this variation because food affects the level of your neurotransmitters—that is, the level of chemicals transmitted to your brain.

Here's how it works. It is midafternoon and you feel extremely anxious. What do you do? You eat. When you eat, you feel an almost immediate stress reduction. However, you will also discover that the relief (which is a reward) is only temporary.

Drug use has similar effects on users. When people use cocaine, they press their gas pedal to the floor. Tranquilizers cause other transmitters to slow the flow, and the user relaxes. Cigarettes and alcohol may have a calming (or brake-pedal) effect. Food is just as powerful as any drug. And like a drug, food affects your emotions and your behavior. Or another way to say it is that food as well as drugs manipulate your transmitters.

Sixth, you are different. By now you may already realize that some chemicals give you no positive response. You may say, "I like the feeling alcohol gives me, but I sure don't like the feeling I get after taking something containing codeine. That prescription drug makes me sicker, or I just feel goofy."

If drugs containing codeine work for some people, why not for you? The answer is simple. Each person's neurochemistry is different. And every person responds differently to various chemicals. Your best friend may drink vodka at night because "I get a nice buzz" from it. You try vodka, and it does nothing for you except give you a hangover headache the next morning. Perhaps it even nauseates you. Your friend gets a reward from vodka, but you don't. This principle is just as true with food as it is with alcohol or drugs.

You have a highly individualized system. Whatever drug

you like, you like it because you get a chemical release in the form of a reward. If you take an aspirin and it relieves your headache, the absence of pain is your reward. If you drink a cup of coffee and feel a temporary surge of energy, that is your reward.

Seventh, your rewards affect your transmitters. For example, if you are stressed and you eat, two things happen. Number one, it affects your neurotransmitter (you pull back on the gas pedal or push it down). Number two, you get rewarded. That is, you liked the response (the feeling) you received from eating, which is a reward. The combination is a reinforcing experience. If you get both benefits, you are apt to repeat this form of behavior. If you liked the feeling you got from eating a certain food, you will eat that food more often and possibly in larger amounts. That is how most addictions start.

Before you finish reading *The Help Yourself Love Yourself Nondiet Weight Loss Plan,* you will learn that various forms of behavior give you both responses, although in different forms. A behavior, chosen properly, will be healthy and offer a long-term benefit. You will learn a behavior other than eating, one that will give you a reward. It then replaces food as your reward.

If you constantly release brake-pedal chemicals, your body will begin to feel out of balance. Although you may feel better emotionally, this excess of neurochemicals is not normal for your body. To get back into balance, enzymes cause the brake-pedal chemicals to have less of an effect, thereby causing physiological balance. Since that doesn't feel good to your emotions, you need to release more brake-pedal chemicals to cause the same effect. This same system works with gas-pedal chemicals.

Suppose you weren't hungry, but you ate once when you felt sluggish or depressed. Within minutes you felt better. Because you had a positive response, the next time you felt low, you ate. Same results. You might not have noticed, but you were probably eating a little more food and doing it more frequently. Over a period of time the pattern of behavior became normal for you. I call it *enzyme adaptation.* Later in this book, I'll show you how to manipulate (or readapt) your enzymes in a healthy way.

You will undergo a neurohormonal change if you use food

for reasons other than to satisfy hunger AND you use it repeatedly to meet those needs AND you use it for an extended period of time.

Neurohormonal change refers to hormones in the brain, and these hormonal changes affect your moods. Even after you have lost weight and have stopped overeating, you have mood swings. Your brain is not yet balanced chemically.

Let's say you have dieted successfully, changed your style of eating, and done all the other things I recommend in this book. Four months later, you still struggle with depressive moods. "Things in my life just don't feel right," you say. Your neurohormones are not yet balanced. For many individuals, this period lasts up to six months, and for a few, as long as a year.

I don't want to discourage you; I just want to prepare you for what lies ahead. You can win over the neurohormonal effects. This book helps you set up your own program to maximize neurohormonal changes.

Eighth, let's look at this information in view of diet recovery. I've already referred to rather complex aspects of brain chemistry, reward centers, neurotransmitters, enzymes, and hormones. When you are food dependent, you have adversely altered all of them. Once your brain has gotten used to using food as a drug because of your overeating and you discontinue your overeating, you will have to retrain your brain. That is, you will have to do something else instead of eating if you want to get the same effects you received from food.

The replacement will have to produce similar effects. *That's crucial to your diet recovery.* This principle also explains why every diet you went on eventually led to failure.

Pause for a minute to rethink all your past dieting experiences. While you followed the program of what to eat (and what not to eat), you stopped overeating. You lost weight. *And then what happened?* Successful dieters—those who lose weight and keep it off for at least five years—know the secret. They diet to lose the weight, but they also change their lifestyle. Instead of taking that next step, you went back to your former way of eating and soon regained your weight.

Gerald is a ten-year member of Weight Watchers. He likes to weigh 190 pounds. He weighs that amount only after he rigorously diets and remains faithful to Weight Watchers.

One time, when he had slimmed from 233 to 196 and was talking about "only 6 pounds to go," I asked him, "Gerald, what are you going to do when you reach 190?"

"I've been thinking about that," he said. "I've just about decided that I'm going to have two pieces of pecan pie."

Gerald didn't learn anything from his diet, except how to lose weight and then put it back on.

Vivian lost forty pounds ten years ago and has kept them off. "I decided," she said, "that along with losing weight, I was going to make serious changes in my life. I set up a simple exercise program. I read a dozen books about developing a positive outlook on life. It worked for me."

Vivian made positive changes on her own, and I commend her. Unfortunately, she's the exception. Most people need help. That's why I've written this book—to help you help yourself.

It comes down to making choices beyond slavishly following a diet that restricts your food intake in some form. Once you lose the weight you want, do you want to start adding pounds again? Or are you willing to work hard at making changes so that you won't have to be food dependent again? The information in this book offers you freedom. That's why I've explained the complexity of your brain. I want you to know what's happening while it's happening.

After stopping any diet, you will do one of three things.

1. You will follow a new life-style (sometimes called behavior modification) that gives you the same reward you received when you were food dependent. That is the goal of this book.

2. You will return to your food dependency. You will be worse off than when you started. You will be overweight again, and you will have added depression and discouragement to your emotional vocabulary.

3. You will no longer be food dependent, but you will transfer your unsatisfied needs to another dependency that will give you a similar effect. Let's say you ate compulsively because your personality sought the high feeling—that is, you pushed down on the gas-pedal neurotransmitter. Your enzymes adapted. Without being aware of what was going on in your body, you *had* to ingest more and more food. If you didn't understand the adaptation of the enzymes, you were aware only that you craved food or certain types of food. You ate, and

yet within an hour, you felt ravenously hungry again. And you continued to add the pounds.

Now you decide to stop the cycle, lose weight, and take up running. If you stick with your program, instead of running two miles you increase the distance to four. No longer content to run three days a week, you run every day or complain, "I just don't feel right if I don't run." Over a period of time, you stop enjoying the exercise, but you keep running anyway.

Congratulations! You have become a compulsive runner. You have successfully transferred your addiction from food dependency to running. You get the same effect (reward) from running that you once got from food.

Are you healthier? Do you feel better about yourself and about your life? I can tell you that the answer is no. Here's why: When you are involved in a compulsive behavior of any kind—eating, drinking, exercising, working—the behavior controls you. It becomes the center of your life. Everything else in your life begins to revolve around your addiction.

Before you started to run, you were overweight and compulsive. Now you are thin and compulsive. But you haven't changed how you feel. You're still subject to depression and feelings of inadequacy and helplessness. *You are a compulsive person* who no longer overeats. You eliminated one form of addiction and transferred it to another form. The effects are the same.

But you don't have to give up. Later in this book, you're going to answer questions to evaluate your neurochemistry. Once you have gone through that questionnaire, you will be able to look at any behavior you have modified. When you ask, "Is this activity good for me?" you can know the answer. If you get a negative answer, you will also know how to turn it into an activity that will be positive.

────────────   ♥ ♥ ♥   ────────────

A vital fact about myself: I commit myself to changing my brain chemistry so that I am free from food dependency.

────────────   ♥ ♥ ♥   ────────────

7

♥

Fixing Your Head

"C'mon, Joel," he said, "food is food. Drugs are drugs. Now I suppose you're going to tell me that I can go on a three-day drunk if I mix my food in the wrong combinations?"

My friend was kidding, of course, but he was struggling to understand the effect of food on the chemicals in the brain. Popular books about diets (including the thousands of diets themselves) say nothing about this issue. Yet food, when broken down in the lab or in the body, shows its chemical makeup.

And as I pointed out in the last chapter, chemicals affect your thoughts and your actions. If you understand that concept, you know that the brain is affected over the years by dieting, misuse of food, bingeing, self-induced vomiting, or mixing food with alcohol and drugs. Now you are ready to figure out what you need to do to change the chemistry in your brain.

Here's a principle to remember:

♥ ♥ ♥

No matter how you feel—
no matter what your energy level—
no matter how compulsive your behavior—
all of this is related to and
controlled by your brain chemicals.

♥ ♥ ♥

"FIX" YOUR NEUROCHEMICALS

I want you to "fix" your neurochemicals so that you can see things clearly and objectively. If your neurochemicals are too low and you're depressed, you'll react negatively. You won't be able to get a reward. At best, you'll set up a goal that says, "A good day is one where I'm not having bad things happen." If your neurochemicals are too high, you'll be so anxious that you'll feel fearful and worried, you'll blow up easily, and you'll have frequent mood swings.

My first goal for you is to help you get your brain chemicals on the right track so that

- you can perceive reality clearly.
- you are motivated to make changes.
- you get rewards from your changes.

You will complete the neurochemical personality evaluation in chapter 8. To get an accurate evaluation, you need to eliminate alcohol, tobacco, drugs, and compulsive behavior, and you need to stop overeating. Be drug-free for at least a week (and that includes drugging yourself through overeating), and then stay drug-free to keep from messing up the chemical balance.

EXAMINE YOUR DIET AND DAILY ACTIVITIES

I want you to look closely at your diet and daily activities. (In later chapters, you'll get more details about your activities.) You can work on changing the chemical mixture in your brain either directly or indirectly. Changing it directly means using a prescribed eating plan and activity program. Changing it indirectly means changing your rewards and selectively altering the way transmission works by your behavior.

To understand how you do that by behavior, please accept this fact: Your behavior or situation can change the chemicals in your brain. Since I don't want to clutter this book with a lot of scientific proof, I hope you will trust me on this point. But I will cite three examples of how behavior and situations interact with thoughts and moods. This is called neurochemical change.

1. At work, the day has been extremely stressful. Your supervisor criticized you publicly, and your coworkers yelled at you. You haven't been doing your most efficient work the past couple of weeks. You've been under stress, and the more stress you feel, the more you think about the situation. Finally, you admit, "I'm not doing things right around here, and I'm not giving it my best." You add guilt to your already bad feelings.

After work, you head for home. You think how much better you'll feel because you can relax and forget the on-the-job problems. But it doesn't work that way. You barely get inside the house, and your spouse says, "We need to talk. You know, you didn't handle this matter right the other day." As you listen to her, you'll explode in anger, or you'll turn silently sullen, depending on how you tend to respond.

No matter what your spouse says, you won't be thinking clearly about the situation. How could you? You're already stressed out. At work, you felt inadequate, maybe even a little worried about keeping your job. Then you come home to relax, but you get more hassles. It's too much to handle.

As your spouse continues, your behavior is affected by everything that has happened the past two weeks. Because you already feel depressed, insecure, and worried, you can't hear clearly. "I'm not in the mood for this," you may say. That's exactly the point. Your mood has been affected by the way you think about what you have been going through.

2. You're planning to host a party, one that is important to you. You have only four more hours to finish cleaning. As the deadline nears, you get more and more anxious. You wonder, *Am I going to get this done in time? What if I'm still cleaning when the first guests arrive?* Your heart pounds, and anxious thoughts fill your mind, which affect your behavior. You become so frantic that you're teary-eyed or angry. You shout at the kids just for walking into the room where you're working.

Why are you feeling this way? Because of your thoughts. The more you think about your unfinished work and the arrival of your guests, the more frantic your behavior becomes (tears and shouts). That is how thoughts affect behavior, which changes neurochemicals.

3. You think you're not a nice person. You didn't just come

up with the idea. You were programmed to think of yourself that way. You might have been the child of an overeater. You were raised in a dysfunctional family. Perhaps you were raised in a cultural situation where the people of your city said that citizens of your ethnic background are not nice people. None of this has to do with whether you are really nice or not, but it's a learned response. If you hear it said often enough or over a long enough period of time that you are not a nice person, your brain stores up the information: "I am not a nice person."

Years later, you are married and have children. You hug your children every day. You do kind things for them. You do all the things that a "nice person" does, but you can't think of yourself that way. Your brain keeps telling you, "I am not nice." Because of your background, this response is automatic—a Pavlovian response.

PAVLOVIAN RESPONSE

Here's what I mean by Pavlovian response. It began with laboratory experiments that showed the effects of repeated behavior, which is called *conditioned reflex* or *conditioned response*. It was the result of the work of Ivan Pavlov, a famous Russian physiologist, who won a Nobel Prize in 1904 for his work on digestion.

Pavlov investigated the secretion of saliva in dogs. He began by ringing a bell just before he fed the dogs. He repeated the process over a period of time until they had been conditioned to expect the food after they heard the bell ring. Later he rang the bell without feeding the dogs, and saliva flowed from their mouths, even though no food was given to them.

Pavlov conditioned the dogs to salivate as if they actually had meat in front of them. Your brain functions the same way. For example, if you ate every time you felt depressed and afterward your mood improved, you became conditioned to using food to lessen your negative feelings. However, if you become depressed and you don't get any food, you're going to have a tremendous craving. You'll feel you have to have it. That's called compulsion. You have programmed your brain to feel a relief of depression when you eat.

Now I want to tell you how to change your Pavlovian responses. I want to help you think about

- yourself.
- your perceptions of life.
- your feelings toward God and others.
- your problems.
- your activities.
- your communication and interaction with others.
- what you eat.

I will show you what will change your neurochemistry, and I will focus on what you eat. What you eat—your daily, habitual style of eating or dieting—affects you in many ways. For one thing, the neurotransmitters in your brain depend on the amino acids from the foods you eat. The conversion of amino acids to neurotransmitters depends on the quality and quantity of amino acids you ingest.

Red meat, such as beef and pork, contains different amino acids from those in poultry or fish. Some people eat red meat and feel more anxiety than those who eat turkey. You may or may not be affected by your choice of red meat or poultry. In the section on eating plans, I'll point out options for you. Try them and if they work by making you feel less food dependent, stay with them. If they don't affect you, you may wish to try a broader-based eating plan.

A MODEL OF BEHAVIOR

Now I want to share with you a way in which we function as people. It is called a model of behavior.

All of us have conflicts. Conflicts create stress in life. When I conduct stress workshops, a few individuals always say, "Dr. Robertson, I came because I want you to help me get rid of my stress."

"The only way you're going to get rid of your stress," I tell them, "is to die. By virtue of being alive, you have stressful situations."

Your purpose isn't to get rid of stress, but it is to eliminate harmful tension or stress that works adversely in your life.

Later I'll discuss where conflicts come from, but right now I want you to think about this fact: *A conflict creates a thought.* That thought could be fear, anger, or a sense of insecurity or inadequacy. Or you could have a positive, happy thought. Regardless of your thoughts, those thoughts change your neurochemistry. That change then affects the way your brain functions.

If you feel happy and contented, you'll probably see the best, most positive aspects of a situation. If you're in a depressed mood, you'll likely see it from the worst perspective. The difference lies in the way you think about any situation.

Your chemistry change creates an emotional response. That response may be stress, anxiety, or depression. Generally, you aren't even aware that you have such thoughts because they happen quickly and almost unconsciously. You don't know about the neurochemicals involved, but you may be aware when you are in a tense or conflicting situation. Or you may not be aware of the stress.

For example, when you were thinking you were not a nice person and yet you hugged your children, you might not have realized you had a conflict. It was conflict because you were being nice while your brain was programmed to tell you that you were not nice. You did something contrary to your belief system. That is the definition of conflict.

Perhaps an illustration will help. Suppose my wife and I disagreed on our vacation plans. That's conflict. I wanted to go to the mountains, and Vickie wanted to visit friends at the lake. When we had the conflict, angry thoughts filled my head. My thoughts then changed the chemicals in my brain, and I became stressed.

I didn't feel the anger. I couldn't admit I was angry because I was taught that good people do not get angry. They control their emotions. I was feeling something negative, and since I couldn't name it as anger, I decided I was feeling stressful. "I feel stress in our relationship," I said to Vickie later, "but I don't know why. Now what do I do?"

Like you, I have four options when I face an emotional response.

1. I can direct my response against myself psychologically. It is psychologically directed at my inner self. That means I put myself down. I say, "Wow, Joel, you are such a rotten person to fight with Vickie. She's always understanding. She's the one who goes where you want to go for vacation. Why does she always have to give in? You're a mean, selfish person even

to want to go to the mountains." My thoughts attack who I am. I tear down my self-esteem.

2. I can direct my response against myself physically. I may then develop a stomachache, ulcers, or high blood pressure, or I may come down with the flu. As you may know, many major diseases such as cancer and heart ailments are related to prolonged stress.

3. I can blame somebody else. In this case, Vickie is the logical one. I think, *Vickie is just being selfish. She knows I prefer the mountains. We saw her friends three years ago at the lake. We can go to the lake anytime.*

4. I can accept that I have the response. Once I say, "Hey, Joel, you're really feeling some tension here," I can go back to the conflict with Vickie. "Look, let's start again," I can say to her. "We need to talk about this some more." This approach is healthy.

Most of us don't recognize that we have directed our response against ourselves psychologically or physically or blamed others, but we turn to some form of behavior to take care of the emotion. That behavior can be spouse abuse, child abuse, alcohol or drug abuse, problem avoidance, overeating, compulsive cleaning, gambling, shopping, or spending money. It's a behavior that is done consistently and automatically.

Whatever behavior I choose in my conflict gives me a chemical reward; I normalize the unbalanced chemical. Whatever I do gives me temporary relief.

Let's go through this again in sequential steps.

1. When my wants differed from those of my wife, the result was conflict.
2. My conflict produced chemical changes that resulted in my feeling anger.
3. Because I could not admit I was angry, I decided I was feeling stress.
4. I directed my emotion (anger) at Vickie by blaming her for the conflict.
5. Because I blamed Vickie for the conflict, I was rid of my anger.
6. Temporarily, my neurochemicals normalized, and my anger went away.
7. I felt great—for the moment anyway.

If the incident had actually happened, I would probably
have said in Step 4: "I'll just forget it." I wouldn't really forget
it; I would eat a candy bar. The next time I had a conflict with
Vickie, I would reach for candy. The form of behavior worked.
It might not have been the best choice, and it certainly wasn't
the only choice. But because it relieved the tension without
causing me discomfort, I'll tend to use food the next time I
encounter a similar situation.

Sometimes in seminars I ask, "What behavior gives you
comfort? You've just had one of the worst days of the year.
Absolutely everything went wrong. What will reward you?
That is, what will make you feel better?"

I get a variety of answers:

- "Have two beers."
- "Smoke a cigarette."
- "Go shopping and spend a lot of money."
- "Clean the house—every room, every spot."
- "Just go to bed with the blinds drawn and the tele-
  phone unplugged."
- "Go to the best restaurant in town and treat myself
  to the most expensive meal on the menu."

Then I turn the situation around and say to the same people, "You have just had one of the best days of your life.
Absolutely everything went right. How do you celebrate?"

I usually get the same answers—alcohol, cigarettes, shopping, drugs, and food.

To understand this, go back to Pavlov and his model of
conditioned response. He rang the bell, and the dogs salivated,
even when there was no food. Once you have a thought that is
caused by conflict, your neurochemicals change, resulting in
an emotional response that causes you *automatically* to turn to
your accustomed behavior. It is so automatic, I can state it this
way: You do something that is beyond your control. You reach
for the candy bar. It doesn't matter if you have already eaten
fifteen candy bars or just finished a gourmet meal. If a new
conflict arises, you do what you have become programmed to
do.

Years ago I heard the actress Geraldine Fitzgerald talk
about her once-heavy smoking habit. She said that whenever

the telephone rang, she *had* to have a cigarette in her hand before she could concentrate on the conversation. That was the hardest part of the smoking habit for her to break—lighting up at the ringing of the phone.

If you realize that you reach for the candy bar under stress, you probably promise yourself that you will stop. You really want to stop, too. But you don't. You look at the candy and say to yourself, "I don't want to eat when I feel this way." But you feel helpless (and you are!). When you get into a conflict that causes the particular chemical change and emotional response, you know only one behavior—you must eat. The bell has rung, so your response to eat is beyond your control as much as salivating was to the dogs. It has become a physiological response. If you manage to resist eating, or if you have no food available, you feel miserable, agitated, depressed, or extremely angry.

Obviously, if you could figure out how to keep the bell from going off, you could overcome compulsive eating. That is exactly where I intend to lead you. Before you complete this book, you will learn how to silence the bell that makes you eat.

But there's more to it than that. You will still have bells ringing from other conditioned situations—we all do. You can learn to anticipate the bells before they go off. If you do that, you can respond differently to conflict. Your chemicals will change, and you can teach yourself to respond automatically in a different fashion.

Five years ago some acquaintances came to us and said, "We have friends who are moving away. They own a seven-year-old German shepherd they can't take with them. She's beautiful. We're trying to help them find a good home for the animal. Would you take her?"

Once they assured us that the dog was house-trained, we said, "Bring her over." When we saw the dog, we decided to keep her. That evening, the dog whined to go outside. I thought the best thing to do initially was to put her on a leash and walk with her. We have a lot of land, and she didn't know the area.

I went over to hook the leash on her collar. The dog hit the floor and began shaking, quivering, and trying to crawl away. I pulled back and stared at her: "Why are you terrified of me?"

I shook my head and backed off. Immediately, the hundred-pound dog was fine again. Vickie, who had watched the bizarre happening, took the leash and started toward the dog. The animal actually walked toward Vickie!

It didn't take a dog psychologist to realize that the German shepherd had been mistreated or beaten by a *man*. Today I can walk up to this dog, and she still flinches and looks away. I have made progress. She lets me pet her. She no longer tries to crawl away.

As you think about your problem with food, I can tell you that you won't stop your automatic behavior. You may still flinch, but you can gain control. That's what you can expect and work toward. Whenever you feel stress accelerating, you may hear the voice in your head say, "Just a quick snack. Not much, but enough to take off the edge..." That's what I mean by the "flinch." But you will recognize it for what it is. You will be able to choose your response to the call to eat.

───────── ♥ ♥ ♥ ─────────

Vital facts about myself: I have learned automatic responses to food. I can change those responses. I am changing those responses.

───────── ♥ ♥ ♥ ─────────

8

— ♥ —

Your Neurochemical Personality

We all get rewarded in different ways. If I want to relax, I choose to run, climb mountains, or go white-water rafting. I choose activity-oriented exercises because I get a reward from excitatory or gas-pedal neurochemicals.

On the other hand, many people relax by watching television or reading a book. They relax by using their inhibitory or brake-pedal neurochemicals. However, if you want to see me stressed, ask me to read or watch television for an extended period of time. To a point, stress is comfortable for me. I enjoy having a little bit of stress, but I dislike depression. Because I like stress only a little, I enjoy not having long business meetings or lengthy periods of nonactivity relaxation. I start feeling restless, and if nothing happens to get me out of the situation, I become irritated.

You may be the opposite type, and you prefer to experience a little depression rather than get too excited. If that's the case, you may be somewhat of a perfectionist or someone who needs to be in control. You then work to make sure there are no curve balls thrown into your life because you don't like a high level of anxiety. You'd rather be a little bit bored and depressed.

Earlier I said that in your brain you have gas-pedal chemicals and brake-pedal chemicals. People get a reward by pushing down on the gas pedal (going fast), or they can get the same effect by releasing or pulling back on the brake pedal. They are the *arousal personalities*. Still other people get a reward by pushing down on the brake pedal, and some by releasing or letting up on the gas pedal. They have *satiation personalities*. Some individuals are a combination of the two.

arousal personality: a neurochemical personality type that enjoys or is more comfortable with excitatory thoughts, activities, or behavior

satiation personality: a neurochemical personality type that is more comfortable with or prefers a decrease in neurotransmission (for most people, overeating has a quieting effect)

Don't think of either neurochemical personality as right or wrong, good or bad. The way you react has to do with the chemical makeup in your brain. It is just one way of helping you understand who you are.

By the way, if you are an arousal personality—if you like gas-pedal living—you probably aren't good at following a diet very long. However, if you have a satiation personality—you are brake oriented—you love diets and do extremely well in following them.

You should understand enough about yourself to know what you will do and what you won't do. You should know whether you respond well to groups or do better in one-to-one situations. You start with learning what type of behavior rewards you.

Two sisters illustrate the personality types. Anne and Sarah grew up in a dysfunctional home. Their father weighed more than 300 pounds before he underwent a stomach bypass. His weight now hovers around 230. His closet contains four different sizes of clothes; the largest pants have a waist of fifty-four inches, and the smallest have a forty-inch waist.

Anne and Sarah's mother is a yo-yo dieter. She is thirty-five pounds overweight at her maximum, and at her lowest point she gets down to just under the figure given as the national medium weight for her height.

Anne turns to food constantly. She wouldn't leave the house without a supply of snack food inside her purse. She is slightly overweight, and people marvel at her energy level. She can start the day out earlier than anyone else and keep going until everyone else drops. She is the family member who gets things done.

By contrast, Sarah is quiet and thin. Her family does not

know that she is a purger. She eats large meals and then induces vomiting at least once every other day. Although she is the only member of the family who is not overweight, she tells no one her secret.

Both sisters have food-dependency problems, but they have different neurochemical personalities. Anne has an *arousal neurochemical personality* because she moves with energy and tackles projects that keep her stirred up, excited, and stimulated. Sarah, however, is a *satiation neurochemical personality*. She seeks calmness and security. Sarah never speaks unless someone initiates the conversation. "I'd like to melt into the floor sometimes," she says, "especially when Anne and my parents get into their big arguments."

Anne's and Sarah's personality types depend on what they respond to in the neurochemical reward center. Anne isn't superior to Sarah or Sarah to Anne. Because of their distinct individuality, they respond differently to life.

Here are definitions of both types, taken from *Help Yourself*.

The Arousal Personality

The arousal personality is excitement oriented, preferring feelings of excitement or "gas-pedal" neurochemical release. These personalities prefer a fast pace over relaxation and boredom. To relax, such personalities must do something to make them feel good. They may enjoy cross-country skiing, diving, swimming, running, and other action-oriented activities. They are more prone to developing addictions to gambling, sex, risk taking, and drugs. They will be attracted to emotional-oriented churches, exercise programs, and changes that provide release of excitatory neurochemicals. They are afraid of being depressed, being alone, and having nothing to do. Often, if things are going fine, they will create a problem to solve. Anxiety and stress are more comfortable to them than boredom or depression.

The Satiation Personality

The satiation personality is antianxiety oriented and enjoys the feeling of relaxation or "brake-pedal" neurochemical release. The mellowing out and self-reflecting spirit means these personalities enjoy relationship activities more than action-oriented activities. They are prone to food, media fascination (especially TV), relationship, perfection, and control addictions. They are so afraid of anxiety, they often become perfectionists and controllers to ward off change or to stop changes from causing anxiety. For them, boredom is more comfortable than excitement.

Most people are a combination of needs, but they generally show a preference for one or the other. This preference is most evident when they feel out of balance or when things "aren't quite right."

Once you are aware of your neurochemical personality, you can use that information to learn four important things:

1. What works in your recovery.
2. What you unconsciously resist.
3. Whether your style of food dependency is consistent with your personality.
4. Which specific activities reward you or cause you to feel good.

YOUR NEUROCHEMICAL PERSONALITY

To learn your neurochemical personality, answer the twenty-four questions with yes or no. If you're not certain, use yes if it is generally true. Please answer every question.

1. Do you choose activities that require active participation?   Yes ☐   No ☐

2. Do you choose activities in which you passively participate or watch the active participants?   Yes ☐   No ☐

3. Are you comfortable socializing with large groups of people?   Yes ☐   No ☐

4. Have you ever had any trouble with the police when you were involved in your preferred activities?   Yes ☐   No ☐

5. Do you enjoy watching movies in which violence and action dominate?   Yes ☐   No ☐

6. Do you like to gamble?　Yes ☐　　No ☐

7. Do you buy lottery tickets or bet on sporting events?　Yes ☐　　No ☐

8. Do you prefer to attend social gatherings that include food? Before agreeing to attend, do you check to make sure refreshments of some kind will be served?　Yes ☐　　No ☐

9. Do you enjoy eating the kind of meal where you leave the table with an increased energy level?　Yes ☐　　No ☐

10. Do you feel good when you engage in risk-oriented activities (such as speeding, mountain climbing, hang gliding, racing)?　Yes ☐　　No ☐

11. When you feel stressed, do sexual activities relax you and lessen the stress?　Yes ☐　　No ☐

12. Do you participate in groups (including religious groups) that have strong beliefs and require your emotional involvement?　Yes ☐　　No ☐

13. Do you like intimate, close communications with small groups?　Yes ☐　　No ☐

14. Do you continue to eat even after you are full?　Yes ☐　　No ☐

15. Do you eat when you are depressed, anxious, or angry?　Yes ☐　　No ☐

16. Do you use food, alcohol, or drugs when you want to relax?　Yes ☐　　No ☐

17. Do you like drugs that decrease your anxiety (including prescription medication)?　Yes ☐　　No ☐

18. Do you try to find ways to avoid conflict?　Yes ☐　　No ☐

19. Do you watch more than fifteen hours of television a week?　Yes ☐　　No ☐

20. Do you attend movies or watch movies on TV at least twice weekly?　Yes ☐　　No ☐

21. Do you rent videotapes at least once a week?   Yes ☐   No ☐

22. When depressed, do you participate in sexual activities to increase your energy?   Yes ☐   No ☐

23. Do you participate in groups (including religious groups) that have strict ethics, rules, or codes of behavior?   Yes ☐   No ☐

24. Do you spend much of your free time alone?   Yes ☐   No ☐

Scoring

1. Add your "yes" answers for 1 through 12 and put the total here: _____

2. Add your "yes" answers for 13 through 24 and put the total here: _____

If you had more "yes" answers to questions 1 through 12, you are an arousal personality. If you had more "yes" answers to 13 through 24, you are a satiation personality. If you have equal numbers of "yes" answers and "no" answers, read the description of each personality and choose the one you believe describes you more correctly.

I AM A/AN _____ PERSONALITY.

♥   ♥   ♥

This information is crucial for your recovery. Your choices of social activities, physical activities, eating plans, therapy, and support options relate to your reward center type.

YOUR BASELINE NEUROTRANSMISSION LEVELS

Next, you need to identify your baseline neurotransmission levels as part of the necessary information to set up your program of recovering from food dependency. *Baseline neurotransmission* is a term that refers to what your brain considers the normal flow of chemicals.

To figure out your baseline neurotransmission levels, you

first need to consider genetic and generational factors. If your baseline neurotransmission level is caused by genetics or generational levels, your recovery will focus on changing the neurochemical levels. If your food dependency changed your baseline neurotransmission level, you will need to adapt your behavior.

1. Genetic or Generational Influences

The following questions can assist in determining if your food dependency has genetic or generational influences. As before, answer yes or no to each question.

1. Does/did your biological father have a food-related problem?   Yes ☐   No ☐

2. Does/did your biological mother have a food-related problem?   Yes ☐   No ☐

3. Does/did two or more of your biological grandparents have food-related problems?   Yes ☐   No ☐

4. Does/did two or more of your biological siblings have food-related problems?   Yes ☐   No ☐

5. Does/did one or more of your biological children have food-related problems?   Yes ☐   No ☐

Total Yes＿＿＿＿＿＿   Total No＿＿＿＿＿＿

"Yes" answers to two or more questions indicate the presence of generational or genetic influences. Four or more "yes" answers indicate that genetic or generational influences play a primary role in your addictive process. Your recovery will certainly require neurochemical manipulation through various techniques.

2. Acquired Influences

An acquired imbalance comes from consistent, long-term behavior. It happens when you constantly overeat, are a chronic dieter, or are a purger or an anorexic. The following questions will assist you in deciding if your food-dependency problem is acquired. Answer yes or no to each question.

1. Have you done this behavior at least three times weekly for at least six months?   Yes ☐   No ☐

2. Have you felt more depressed or in a "low" mood since you became aware that you had a food-related problem?   Yes ☐   No ☐

3. Have you felt more anxiety or nervousness since you became aware that you had a food-related problem?   Yes ☐   No ☐

4. Whenever you stopped overeating or giving in to your food-related behavior, did your depression increase?   Yes ☐   No ☐

5. Whenever you stopped overeating or giving in to your food-related behavior, did your anxiety increase?   Yes ☐   No ☐

Total Yes _____   Total No _____

A "yes" answer to two or more questions indicates the addiction or behavior has changed your baseline neurochemical level. It is common to have genetic alterations and acquired alterations at the same time. The genetic influences created the addiction, while the behavior continued to alter them.

Neurotransmission Levels

The term *neurotransmission level* refers to the level at which the chemicals in your brain are transmitted. The baseline level is what your brain thinks is normal, although it may not be. It isn't necessarily what feels good, but what your body needs.

The following questions will help you determine whether your baseline neurotransmission level is deficient or excessive. Answer yes or no to each question.

1. When you're quiet and inactive, do you frequently feel sad or depressed?   Yes ☐   No ☐

2. Do you think of your life as exciting and vibrant?   Yes ☐   No ☐

3. Do you participate in activities that involve excitement, physical challenge, and adventure?   Yes ☐   No ☐

4. Do you frequently procrastinate or lack motivation to do little things that you know need doing?   Yes ☐   No ☐

5. Do you put too much energy or commitment into one or two areas of your life?   Yes ☐   No ☐

6. When you want to relax, do you often feel hyper or "wired"?   Yes ☐   No ☐

7. Do little things upset you, and then you start to feel depressed?   Yes ☐   No ☐

8. Do little things frequently upset you and cause you to feel anxious?   Yes ☐   No ☐

9. Do your anxieties worsen when you're under stress?   Yes ☐   No ☐

10. Do you often find it difficult to concentrate on your job or important issues?   Yes ☐   No ☐

Downer Questions

Count the number of "yes" answers from questions 1, 4, 7, 8, and 10. _____

Upper Questions

Count the number of "yes" answers from questions 2, 3, 5, 6, and 9. _____

If you answered yes to more Downer Questions, your neurotransmission is probably deficient, too.

If you answered yes to more Upper Questions, your neurotransmission is probably excessive.

If you answered yes to the same number of Downer and Upper Questions, you probably have no preference in neurotransmission.

♥ ♥ ♥

Genetic and generational alterations require neurochemical corrections to help in behavioral changes. Diet, exercise, and behavioral options (coming up later in this book) can help. If you follow them, you can also focus on spiritual and behavioral changes.

If your addiction is acquired, spiritual and behavioral changes may receive the first emphasis, followed by diet and exercise.

If you're serious about recovery, begin these programs within a month.

The most difficult task in developing a recovery plan is to figure out your baseline neurotransmission level. For most individuals, a few questions are enough to make this determination.

After you've answered the questions in this section, you may want a neurochemical evaluation if your findings aren't clear. For further information on neurochemical evaluations, write or phone: The Robertson Institute, Ltd., 3555 Pierce Road, Saginaw, MI 48604, (517) 799-8720.

9

— ♥ —

Themes of Life

MAJOR THEMES

Food dependency involves the issues I've mentioned, and it also includes themes. My use of the word *themes* refers to a psychological need. Perhaps the following definitions will help you understand the difference between theme and addiction.

theme: a psychological need

addiction: the method used to satisfy that need

For example, a person's theme could be a need for acceptance. He or she might satisfy the need by becoming addicted to prescription drugs. In one sense, the addiction you choose is secondary. Because of your unique personality, you gravitate toward the forms of addictive behavior that will satisfy your need. If you concentrate on cutting out the addiction, you don't get to the real issues in your life. If you have a bullet lodged in your leg, you can concentrate on stanching the flow of blood (the symptom), or you can take the bullet out because it causes the loss of blood.

Addiction and compulsive behavior work the same way. Because of who you are, you have chosen food as your way to satisfy needs of which you may not even be fully aware. If you concentrate only on the food issue, all you need to do is try a new diet. And what happens? Once you finish the diet, you start over again putting the weight back on.

But if you look at your themes—the problems underlying your need to depend on food—you can overcome the problem. That may also explain to you the reason I said previously that it takes work to become free from your food dependency.

Do you remember the story about my two Shetland ponies? The solution to cleaning up the barn was to start with *one* filled pitchfork. I tossed it out. Then I went back to the pile and lifted up more. I continued, going down to the next layer. That's the opposite of how diets work. Diets stay on the top layer and never get down to the bottom. They are teaching you to keep working on the top layers, and you never even get around to thinking about closing the barn door.

You reach toward the bottom layer when you start accepting your themes—your basic needs. Like everyone else, you have one or more themes in your life. Your themes motivate you, push you, and make you get things done. The themes (needs) gnaw at you until you make changes based on satisfying those themes. Or you just give up and feel hopeless.

Later in this chapter, I'll take you through a step-by-step exercise to enable you to discover your theme (or themes). Then I'll show you how to make sensible changes. These changes are sensible because they work toward meeting your basic needs instead of helping you deny or fight them.

For now, I want to give you a list of themes that I have found most common among the individuals who have come to see me. As you read, you may identify yours.

1. Adequacy

If this is your theme, you work hard to feel effective and competent. You set yourself up, unconsciously of course, to fail. Then you can say, "See, I knew I would fail."

I know a gifted athlete who is now in his late forties. Although he once achieved success on the field, he constantly fails at business. He all but signs contracts for endorsements and then does something to offend the sponsors. He is not aware of his inadequacy, and he blames "those people" who hinder him.

If this is your theme, you may accomplish something that you assume almost anybody could do. You get no reward and no sense of accomplishment. You then continue to follow a theme of inadequacy.

One of the most devastating diseases in society today is the feeling of inadequacy. The compulsion to acquire possessions, money, prestige, and control comes from these feelings of inadequacy. If you feel inadequate or insecure, you may attempt to make the exterior of your life appear successful. It is your way to compensate for the lack of peace on the inside. No matter how outwardly successful you are or how talented, your accomplishments don't matter if you don't like yourself.

You may show signs of giving up, or you behave as if nothing really matters. You don't set goals. "Why should I?" you say to yourself. "I'm just going to fail anyway." You settle into a life of apathy. "That's all there is," you tell yourself in your misery.

2. Approval Seeking

Approval through eating is usually linked to mother-child relationships. If I eat everything on my plate, Mom will think I like her and I am a good person. This theme continues with your spouse. You even transfer it to other relationships so that you work very hard to please others.

Healthy approval seeking is a natural human characteristic. Who doesn't want to be liked and appreciated? Approval seeking becomes a theme when you sacrifice your beliefs, values, and opinions to get that approval.

Some individuals seem confident and speak up boldly so that few would accuse them of seeking approval. However, by listening closely, I've noticed that they don't state opinions—they present their opinions as facts, which is evidence of their insecurity. Since no one can reasonably argue against facts, they push away rejection. Their insecurity and fear of rejection sometimes cause them to be labeled know-it-alls.

3. Pleasure

Some people just love to eat. The pleasure is in eating and overindulging. They don't know when to quit.

You may defend this behavior by saying, "I deserve everything that I get. I deserve pleasure all the time, and I don't want responsibility."

Pleasure themes show themselves if you seek to feel good from recreation and sexual activities. Recreation as a form of relaxing is popular today and usually healthy. The pleasure theme becomes an issue when bowling, golf, or video and computer games take the place of interaction with the family. Overeating can directly relate to a search to feel good—a theme of pleasure.

4. Power

Ever look at yourself and say, "I'm really looking for power"? Probably not, but it may be one of your themes.

Often people overeat and diet for control. (And control is a form of power!) Your life may be so out of control that dieting offers you at least one area in your life where you have a certain amount of domination. Your mind interprets this control as power. Power has been a major theme for many, accompanied by the drive for more money or a better position. In fact, it has become our society's standard for defining success.

The power theme is identified rather easily by other people. Outsiders usually observe (and may even tell you), "Your need to be in charge seems more important than your family, friends, or job."

Of course, if you have a power theme, you won't want to acknowledge such information. That's your defense system at work.

If power is your theme, it is probably directed toward accumulating money, getting a better position, controlling others, enhancing your physical appearance, or emphasizing your intellectual ability or education. If you focus on success by achieving high positions, getting large amounts of money, being recognized for your intelligence, or being labeled handsome or beautiful, you are caught up in a power theme.

Your power theme becomes a serious problem when you seek to have your needs met at the expense of others. While you are climbing the company ladder out of your need for power, you tend to

- neglect your children.
- have no energy to enjoy your spouse.
- be unable to relax with friends.
- complain about how much work you have to do and the responsibility you carry.

Such behavior indicates power is your theme.

5. Recognition

If you are overweight, you're easily recognized. You also may control family systems and cause the family to revolve around you and your needs. Instead of recognizing this tendency, you interpret yourself as being the glue that bonds the family together. Since you get what you want, you are then recognized as the one who holds the family together.

Although everyone needs to be recognized, appreciated, and respected, the difficulty comes if your life revolves around this need. You calculate your actions so that others will applaud what you do. Internal recognition isn't enough because you need approval and recognition of your good deeds, which must come from other people.

When you do something for others, you want the world to know. You probably find a way to tell them, too. You serve from a desire not to help but to look good and to be recognized as a caring person. You brag or even exaggerate your accomplishments.

6. Responsibility Avoidance

Being overweight is not being responsible to your family, your health, and yourself. Overeating may be a form of rebellion that allows you to avoid social situations and being with others. "After all," you may be saying on some unconscious level, "if I'm overweight, who is going to ask me to go bike riding or...?"

Being responsible infringes on selfish human nature. Selfishness makes doing for others a chore and creates anger and frustration. Society promotes selfishness with catchy phrases such as, "Look out for number one."

Many times I've heard people speaking of feeling responsible, and somebody quickly speaks up to set them straight, "You're responsible only for yourself," or "Just do your own thing." A few popular therapists have chided people for feeling responsible, sometimes implying it's a weakness (or even a sickness) to feel committed to others.

You may be avoiding responsibility by refusing to get involved. You back off from

- making career goals and commitments.
- obligating yourself to help the needy.

- volunteering at church or civic organizations.
- giving yourself in relationships with others.

Is yours one of those homes where you have shifted from a commitment to each other to a search for selfish fulfillment of individual needs? Are you moving away from family responsibilities by declaring, "I have to live my own life. I have to take care of my needs"?

I don't deny that you need to take care of yourself, but it's easy to use your need as an excuse for selfish living.

MINOR THEMES

I have also observed a few other themes worth noting. They are less common (which is why I call them minor) but every bit as valid.

1. Avoidance

How do you handle problems that confront you? If you hate to face them head-on or find reasons not to cope with them, you avoid the problems. You go along with the old idea, "Problems will go away if you don't think about them." They don't go away. You just continue to evade situations.

2. Nonacceptance

You don't find it easy to accept other people or ideas that differ from your own. You tend to categorize everything as either wrong or right with no other options possible.

In some churches, I've heard individuals say, "This is what the Bible says. This is what the Bible means. That settles it." They seem unable to accept the fact that they may have misinterpreted or misunderstood.

3. Revenge

Maybe you're frustrated with everybody around you. "Why should they have it better than I do?" you ask. Your thoughts often center on getting even, on paying others back for the harm they have done to you.

4. Excitement

The risk taker or thrill seeker must have bigger challenges. You seek dangerous situations.

5. Superiority

You feel you are above others. You take comfort in thinking of yourself as wiser, more intelligent, or more capable than others. Secretly you may smirk or laugh at their stupidity.

♥ ♥ ♥

These are some common themes of people like you who are food dependent. A theme dictates how you react to certain situations and determines why you behave as you do. Because you could never satisfy your themes, you turned to food to be comforted, to "medicate," and to enable you to continue to function. Because your themes deprive you of energy you could use to work with healthy issues, you need to identify them and resolve them.

IDENTIFYING YOUR THEMES

Rodney was a compulsive eater—a man who planned every day's activities around his eating. He ate a "light snack" of yogurt when he got out of bed and then a "hearty breakfast to give me energy for the day." That hearty breakfast included two or three cups of flavored coffee with a heavy sugar-fat content. On his break at the office, Rodney had a Danish and coffee. He kept a jar of hard candy on his desk "to nibble on because I've heard that hard candy isn't as fattening." If he was going to be out of the office, he grabbed small packages of cheese and crackers, working his schedule so that he could have a leisurely lunch while he did business. Sometimes he scheduled a second "power lunch" where he ate "moderately light."

As Rodney continued to tell me about his day, I realized he was never more than an hour away from food. He worked carefully to live that way, although he admitted that it was stressful at times.

Rodney told me that he was aware of some of his emotions:

"I'm always afraid that I won't do a good job. I'm the best in our office if you look at the awards I've won. But I don't seem to be able to rest with what I've done. Every day I have to start proving myself over and over."

After taking my tests, Rodney was able to see his emotions involved his sense of inadequacy, loneliness, and insecurity. We looked at themes, and power headed the list. He learned his real issue was power or the need to get control. As he was able to single out that issue, he was able to change. Previously, he had been confused and didn't know what to fix first.

Rodney learned something important. Like him, you can identify your major themes in life, which will help you eliminate your need for compulsive overeating.

THEMES

The following questions will help you identify your compulsive themes. Answer each question with yes or no. If you are unsure, select the one that is true most of the time.

1. Adequacy

1. Have you been told that you sometimes have unrealistic expectations of others?   Yes ☐   No ☐

2. Do you set up unrealistic demands for yourself?   Yes ☐   No ☐

3. Do you avoid doing things because you're afraid you'll fail or you won't do a good enough job?   Yes ☐   No ☐

4. At your job (or school) do you take criticism and negative comments as personal attacks?   Yes ☐   No ☐

5. Do you often feel insecure?   Yes ☐   No ☐

2. Approval seeking

1. Are you comfortable when others express their opinions before you speak?   Yes ☐   No ☐

2. Do you dress or behave in particular ways to make others accept you more readily?   Yes ☐   No ☐

3. Do you put a lot of effort into being liked?   Yes ☐   No ☐

4. Do you sometimes deny your beliefs so that others will accept you?   Yes ☐   No ☐

5. Is it easier for you to follow than to lead?   Yes ☐   No ☐

3. Pleasure

1. Is it difficult for you to enjoy a quiet evening with friends?   Yes ☐   No ☐

2. Is it common for you to "pay" for entertainment? (This could mean anything from renting videos to paying for sex.)   Yes ☐   No ☐

3. Do family members and friends usually give you what you want?   Yes ☐   No ☐

4. When you have free time, is it important that you use it to have a good time?   Yes ☐   No ☐

5. Do you put off until later important tasks so you can have fun *now*?   Yes ☐   No ☐

4. Power

1. Do you feel that you spend more hours at work than you should?   Yes ☐   No ☐

2. Do you work extremely long hours to make more money, even though you don't have to?   Yes ☐   No ☐

3. In social situations, do you give your opinions on most topics?   Yes ☐   No ☐

4. Are you uncomfortable when persons in authority tell you what to do?   Yes ☐   No ☐

5. Are you a person who needs to be in control of most situations?   Yes ☐   No ☐

5. Responsibility

1. Do you procrastinate often?   Yes ☐   No ☐

2. Does this statement describe you? "I don't volunteer myself to work for organizations or causes because they take up too much time."   Yes ☐   No ☐

3. Does the way you spend your money force you to live from payday to payday?   Yes ☐   No ☐

4. Is it important for you to relax, even when you have many things you need to do?   Yes ☐   No ☐

5. Do you get angry or feel anxious when you are told to do something or you are held responsible if something goes wrong?   Yes ☐   No ☐

6. Recognition

1. Do you work at getting people to respect you?   Yes ☐   No ☐

2. Do you agree to serve on committees that provide high visibility or give you opportunity for more contacts or recognition?   Yes ☐   No ☐

3. Do you normally socialize with people you consider important?   Yes ☐   No ☐

4. Do you buy things to improve your image of being successful, even when that means going into debt?   Yes ☐   No ☐

5. At parties, is most of your conversation related to your work?   Yes ☐   No ☐

♥ ♥ ♥

The element with the greatest number of "yes" answers will indicate your compulsive theme. If several have the same number, discuss the results with your support person and/or group. Ask for input and insight.

Since themes refer to unmet psychological needs, you can't deny them. Your themes are so important, they determine how you react in most situations. They are so habitual, you are probably not aware of your unconscious decisions to have your themes provided for. To overcome your food-dependency problem, you need to know your themes, but you also need to know what in your personality causes you to turn to food when you are in need.

ADDICTIONS

First, let's determine your food-dependency addictions. Once you know your major themes, you are ready to work on the way you have used food to meet those themes. Remember that an addiction is a behavior you do that negatively affects your life. Often other behaviors, in addition to overeating, will be seen in your life.

Look at the following list and determine which addictive behaviors you see in your life. Notice that certain addictions are often associated with a particular theme. We have listed addictions under the themes they are associated with to help you in your evaluation.

Circle the addictions currently present; underline those to which you feel vulnerable.

Power
Activity
Alcohol/drug
Control
Exercise
Gambling
Hypochondria
Intelligence/education
Material
Physical appearance
Rescuing
Risk taking/excitement
Sex
Spending
Stealing
Violence
Work

Adequacy
Activity
Alcohol/drug
Approval seeking
Cleaning
Control
Exercise

Food
Hypochondria
Intelligence/education
Material
Media fascination
Perfection
Physical appearance
Religion
Rescuing
Sex
Stealing
Violence
Work

Pleasure
Activity
Alcohol/drug
Caffeine
Food
Media fascination
Nicotine
Risk taking/excitement
Sex
Violence

Responsibility
Alcohol/drug
Hypochondria
Media fascination
Rescuing
Sex
Stealing

Approval Seeking
Activity
Approval seeking
Cleaning
Exercise
Food
Gambling
Material
Nicotine
Perfection
Religion

Risk taking/excitement
Sex
Spending
Stealing
Violence
Work

Recognition
Activity
Exercise
Gambling
Material
Religion
Risk taking/excitement
Sex
Spending
Stealing
Violence
Work

You may have discovered that you have several addictions within one or two themes. At this stage of your recovery, concentrate on the most prominent addictions and themes. When you work at meeting the needs shown by your themes, your behavior changes. If you find healthy ways to satisfy your themes, you can lay aside unhealthy methods you have used in the past.

MY COMPULSIVE THEME(S) IS/ARE _____

_____

Next, let's classify your addictions. Each addiction should be classified according to whether it satisfies excitatory or inhibitory needs. An excitatory addiction improves moods or relieves depression. An inhibitory addiction decreases anxiety or causes a "mellowing out."

Your addictions will cause your compulsive theme(s) to be excitatory or inhibitory.

MY ADDICTIONS ARE GENERALLY (circle one)
excitatory or inhibitory

In the previous chapter, you decided if you had an excitatory (arousal) or inhibitory (satiation) personality. On page 78, you recorded

I AM A/AN _____ PERSONALITY.

Classifying addictions helps in determining the type of effect you seek. If your neurochemicals are out of balance, you will want to increase or decrease your mood level.

In the pages ahead, you will learn how to use this information to decide on *your* recovery plan, a plan specifically designed for your brain chemistry and addiction.

--------------------- ♥ ♥ ♥ ---------------------

A vital fact about myself: I acknowledge my life themes because they help me win the battle of keeping my weight off.

--------------------- ♥ ♥ ♥ ---------------------

10

— ♥ —

Techniques for Recovery

We can offer a variety of recovery techniques, but deciding on the most effective one for you is essential for successful recovery. When I first use the word *recovery*, some people immediately think of it as a term for alcoholics and drug addicts when they kick their habits. The word has a much wider use. Recovery means

- moving away from the things you do when you are under stress or feel out of balance.
- learning to do the necessary things to maintain neurochemical normalcy.
- identifying your neurochemical profile, your compulsive themes, and your neurotransmission levels.

All of this information moves you toward setting up a program that is built around an eating plan, activities, and behavioral changes and leads to total recovery from food dependency.

IDENTIFYING YOUR NEUROCHEMICAL PROFILE

To discover your most effective method of recovery, you must do the following:

1. Decide if you are an arousal or a satiation personality. (See chapter 8.)
2. Decide if your themes are excitatory or inhibitory. (See chapter 9.)
3. Know your neurotransmission level. To be totally accurate, you need to go to a professional for a neurochemical evaluation. However, most people can develop a plan based on estimated neurotransmission levels. (See chapter 8.)

Refer to your responses in chapters 8 and 9:

- Is your neurochemical personality *satiation* or *arousal*?
- Is your compulsive theme *inhibitory* or *excitatory*?
- Is your neurotransmission level *deficient* or *excessive*?

Find the line across the first three columns in figure 10-1 that matches your findings. The letter in the far right column represents your type of neurochemical profile. For instance, if your neurochemical personality is *arousal*, your compulsive theme is *inhibitory*, and your neurotransmission level is *excessive*, your neurochemical profile is *Type F.*

FIGURE 10-1
Neurochemical Profiles

Neurochemical Personality	Compulsive Theme	Neurotransmission Levels	Neurochemical Profile
satiation	inhibitory	deficient	A
arousal	inhibitory	deficient	B
satiation	excitatory	deficient	C
arousal	excitatory	deficient	D
satiation	inhibitory	excessive	E
arousal	inhibitory	excessive	F
satiation	excitatory	excessive	G
arousal	excitatory	excessive	H

Your neurochemical profile indicates what type of activity, eating plan, or behavioral techniques may be beneficial to you. The profile assists in determining the rewards likely to be most effective over time.

BEHAVIORAL TECHNIQUES

Phil had struggled with obesity most of his life. When his therapist gave him his first assignment, he couldn't believe it. "That's the dumbest thing I ever heard," he said. His therapist wanted him to spend at least one hour a day with friends.

"How can sitting around talking to a bunch of people help me?" he asked.

"For now, just do it," she said.

"Okay," Phil told her with reluctance. He wasn't a social mixer. He went to parties and events and tried to mingle and talk, but he felt ill at ease. At the end of two weeks he came back and reported, "Mingling and mixing with people only made me want to eat more."

Phil got no reward from social mingling. Even so, he tried it because he thought it was important for keeping his weight off and improving his general health. For another six weeks he set up regular social times with his friends. He said, "I never felt anything positive from that, even though a lot of the time they were trying to make me feel supported and cared about." Then Phil added, "And I gained ten pounds."

Being with others is a good idea—for some people. Phil's therapist made the mistake of treating him like others who had come to her. They had profited from the social interaction. Phil was different.

"There I was, just sitting around talking and talking and talking. The others might have had a good time," Phil said, "but I kept thinking of all the time I was wasting."

Changing your behavior is a major part of overcoming food dependencies. Behavior that is consistent with your neurochemistry gives you a reward. It also improves your brain chemistry. In this chapter, you will learn why behavioral techniques are important. Later you will develop your own specific plan based on your neurochemical profile.

I wanted you to know about Phil because he changed through using behavioral techniques.

I offer you a variety of behavioral techniques to help you

- learn the best way to obtain rewards by your chosen form of therapy.
- discover the social situations best for you.
- rethink your spirituality.
- learn whether activity, an eating plan, or medication will be the most significant for you.
- focus on the dynamics that work toward balancing your brain chemicals.
- guide yourself so that you will not need to misuse food.
- keep your thoughts from continuing to change your brain chemistry and create a compulsion to overeat.

You can now concentrate on the proper balance of brain chemistry. Once this happens, no longer will you have thoughts that lead to depression or other negative emotions or situations that cause you to continue overeating. The behavioral recommendations in this chapter are determined by your answers on the neurochemical evaluation (see chapter 8).

You have already examined three factors that determine your neurochemical balance:

1. Your reward center—where you get satisfaction or the lessening of pain.
2. Your themes—which force you to seek rewards.
3. Your imbalanced brain chemicals—which prevent your having a full grasp of reality.

Now you are ready to focus on your behavioral needs. These needs are unique to you, and they revolve around your reward center. As I stated previously, your reward center works on a simple principle: If you do something and find it pleasurable, you'll do it again. If you get nothing out of an activity, you won't repeat it. You are a person with a food-related problem. Obviously, you get something out of overeating, so you continue to misuse food. The purpose of *The Help Yourself Love Yourself Nondiet Weight Loss Plan* is to help you learn other ways to get the same kind of pleasure from sources other than food.

I want to go back to Phil and finish his story. After I examined him and worked with him for one session, he realized that he

- had a Type A profile.
- had themes of power and perfection.
- was a workaholic.

If the therapist had assigned Phil an activity that satisfied his themes and made him feel better about himself, he would more likely have wanted to continue meeting socially with friends.

This is again the principle of the Pavlovian response. The dogs, you recall, responded to the sound of the bell, regardless of whether the researchers produced food. Like them, you're going to "hear" bells going off. They may come from your emotions, your thoughts, or your existing conflicts. When the bells ring, they will force you to do *something*. Right now, you probably overeat. You may also do other forms of behavior of which you're unaware because they are also automatic.

Here's the goal I want you to set for yourself. I want you to find a form of behavior that you can learn to respond to automatically when your bell rings. But it will have to be something that rewards you by making you feel better. If it makes you feel better, you will be less inclined to do negative things.

YOUR THREE PATTERNS

I find it helpful to think of human nature as having three major components: (1) the physical (the body); (2) the emotional (feelings, instincts, and intuition); and (3) the spiritual (the sense of purpose in life and responses to and understanding of God, self, and others).

1. The physical

Activity and exercise are important to get your physical body in shape. But your nerves are part of your emotional as well as your physical makeup. If your nerves are not functioning properly, they will affect the emotions. All three components overlap each other. You need to be aware that the emotional part is tied into the physical part.

2. The emotional

The emotional component carries your moods—which determine whether you're depressed, anxious, irritated, sad, or guilty.

3. The spiritual

This part has more to do with the attitudes, the way you look at who you are, and includes your sense of self-esteem. It involves your innermost being and the person who drives you from a spiritual standpoint. You may be self-oriented, while others are God oriented.

If you are physically ill, your condition will affect you emotionally and spiritually. I hope you will grasp this point because some people cannot develop an emotional wellness or a spiritual wellness until they have taken care of their physical health or well-being.

GETTING HELP AT YOUR ENTRY POINT

Mae is an arthritic with a serious heart condition, diabetes, and hypertension because of her obesity, and she is a survivor of a double mastectomy. She suffers from extreme and chronic pain. "I can't think of a single moment when I'm totally pain-free," she said. Mae has had a difficult time with her spiritual and emotional lives. "I'm in such pain, I can't seem to think about anything else. How can I feel peaceful when my bones ache? How can I praise God when every movement shoots pains through my whole body?"

Obviously, before Mae could do anything about her emotional and spiritual lives, she needed help to get pain-free. The entry point—the place where she started to get help for all three human components—was her physical body. That's what she did. Mae lost eighty-five pounds through a supervised program at the Diet Center. The weight loss alleviated much of her pain. With a change of medication, she now lives with greatly reduced pain.

"You know," Mae said with a genuine smile, "I feel like a real person again." She had begun at the entry point where she needed the most help. Until she did something for her body, nothing could be done for her emotions and her spiritual outlook.

On the other hand, Edward is emotionally ill. He suffers from emotional swings, which is called a bipolar disorder. One day Edward would be morose, depressed, lethargic, and occasionally suicidal. Then, often within hours, he would be a fireball of action and excitement, planning activities, working on projects, and calling people on the phone. Neither condition lasted more than a few days.

Edward finally realized he had a psychiatric illness and received both therapy and medication. Like Mae, once he got help *at his entry point,* he was ready to move on to the other parts of his life. Until then, he had so many mental problems, he couldn't cross over to another area. Either he had no interest in making changes (when he was depressed), or he was convinced that he had solved all his problems when he was euphoric. At neither time did he have an accurate view of his life.

The third part is spiritual illness. Spiritual illness is an unhealthy approach to who you are, how you understand life, and how you see others.

Arthur and Neva were spiritually ill individuals who also had food-dependency problems. Arthur suffered from guilt, unable to believe that God could forgive him. Neva's attitude was that life "has already gone down the tube. Every year life gets more violent, and nothing is fun anymore. Everybody is out to take advantage of me."

If you're spiritually unhealthy, it shows in the way you look at life, yourself, others, and the world around you. Please bear in mind that I'm not referring to theology, denominations, or interpretations of the Bible. *Spiritual* refers to your inner self as well as your relationship with God. When you're spiritually healthy, you are harmonious and integrated, and you understand your strengths. My friend Brian said, "Having spiritual health means treating life positively."

♥ ♥ ♥

Vital facts about myself: I am a physical, emotional, and spiritual being. I accept all of myself.

♥ ♥ ♥

You are a whole person, and your goal is total wholeness. Some things are going to seem fun for you, but others are not. To be "in tune" and healthy, you must consider that the physical, emotional, and spiritual tie together, and you need to work on all three.

The way I respond to a situation or a thought is unique to me. As I think of who I am, my physician told me that I had to follow a prescribed diet, but I probably wouldn't do well. That's because of my personality. The situation would be different if my doctor said, "Joel, if you eat more calories, you're going to have to exercise more."

"No problem," I would assure him. I *want* to exercise more, and I would like to eat more calories.

You may say, "I would rather diet than exercise, so I'll watch my diet to maintain my physical health. Exercising is one of the last things I want to do."

I am right because I am being true to my personality. You are right because you are being faithful to who you are.

When I show you various ways to emotional wellness, remember that one size does *not* fit all. Incorporate only what applies to you. Your point of entry can be through your intellect or emotions. It can be through group activities or individual relationships. You can start your journey by self-reflection. Sometimes you may want to discuss your progress with your support person; at other times you may choose to be alone. There are several ways to emotional health—depending on what works for you.

You can look at your spiritual nature in a variety of ways. Some individuals find their entry through the traditional church setting and a liturgical-type worship. Or you may find that you respond more effectively to a more openly emotional worship experience.

At age twenty-one Daniel asked what he called "the existential questions." He said, "I knew there had to be more to life than what I had experienced. I wanted to know who I was, why I was alive, and what difference my life would make." Daniel had had little religious training, even less interest in the church, and didn't seek to belong to any particular religion. After a year of searching and self-reflection, he became a Christian, but that was not his original goal. His entry point was where he most keenly felt a need.

Now you turn to specific behavioral techniques that are going to be most effective for you. Refer to your neurochemical profile, which you identified earlier in this chapter.

11

— ❤ —

Neurochemical Personalities

Once you have determined your neurochemical profile type, you are ready to learn what recovery techniques will be most effective for you. Certain rewards are likely to be most effective for particular profile types. Find the section treating your profile type in the following material and read it carefully.

TYPE A NEUROCHEMICAL PROFILE

If you have a Type A neurochemical profile, you typically have long-term genetic predispositions to compulsive disorders. An investigation into the family history may reveal alcoholism, perfectionism, compulsive overeating, or other compulsive disorders.

The neurochemical profile suggests the neurochemical baseline or enzyme activity or levels that the brain considers normal may actually be *less* than what would produce good feelings.

There appears to be no behavioral compensation for the altered neurochemistry; that is, you aren't doing exciting activities to overcome the depressed neurotransmission levels. In fact, the low neurotransmission levels may be causing the behavior, which can predispose you to transfer to other addictions.

The goal of Type A neurochemical profiles is to transfer to a positive addiction—initially. Eliminating or minimizing com-

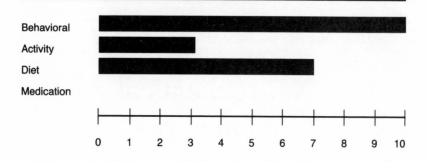

Figure 11-1
Recovery Effectiveness Rating

TYPE A PROFILE

pulsive behavior may be difficult at first. After a period of time, you can eliminate or reduce all compulsive behaviors.

Behavioral changes are the most effective way to obtain rewards and remain consistent with neurochemical needs. I suggest that you read the material in the chapter about behavioral changes and then discuss it thoroughly with members of your support system.

Your need to belong is essential. Without your support system completely behind you, you could hinder the motivation to change. You need support to stay motivated.

Small gatherings or social situations in which you can be self-reflective and receive support would be beneficial. Meditation, Bible studies, self-help, and emotionally supportive activities are probably most acceptable and desirable for you.

You learn spirituality best through a church that emphasizes study. You also interact well with small groups. If forced to share, you may become uncomfortable and stressed.

Activity therapy is beneficial for health, but it's probably more acceptable as a hobby or in a quiet setting instead of with a large group of people.

An eating plan therapy can be most beneficial. You will likely follow it closely.

Negative attitude and frustration may be problems in your recovery process. You have a strong tendency to give up. With your Type A profile, you need to accept yourself and others to maintain the energy to recover.

TYPE B NEUROCHEMICAL PROFILE

If you have a Type B neurochemical profile, you probably have used drugs, alcohol, and/or medication or followed a compulsive behavior—some form of eating disorder—for a long period. You have adapted to the consistent depression of neurotransmitters by generational, environmental, or outside forces, such as diet, drugs, or long-term, consistent behavioral changes. Your enzymatic system has likely adapted to such changes.

There appears to be no behavioral compensation for such altered neurochemistry, and the rewards for behavior appear to be low. Your behavior is probably a result of the altered neurotransmission. Transfer of addiction or compulsion may be low if you monitor your life-style and make changes.

Behavioral changes are important to obtain rewards and remain consistent with your neurochemical needs. Behavioral changes without any consistent activity/exercise program will be less effective than with the activity/exercise program. Group activities or team sports may be more effective than individual activities.

FIGURE 11-2
Recovery Effectiveness Rating

TYPE B PROFILE

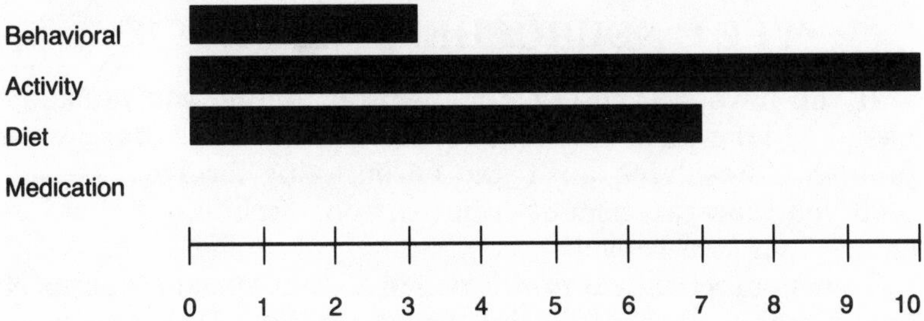

You need independence within the group to enjoy the group process. You tend to be more comfortable knowing what is expected of you than just going along with the group. Self-help fellowships, active involvement in a weight-management program such as the kind offered by Diet Center, and active participation in church activities will be beneficial to you.

Social situations are more comfortable with activities that have some degree of structure. Intellectually or educationally oriented social activities may be most acceptable to you. To be supportive, the family system needs to be aware of the social activities that provide rewards.

You can effectively learn spirituality in a church with a structured environment. Bible studies with intellectual content or emphasis can be helpful. If there is too much emotion involved, you may resist change.

Activity and exercise therapy is essential for your emotional and neurochemical needs as well as for physical health. Activities that make you feel better about yourself while you interact in relationships are extremely valuable. Doing activities with the family, such as skiing or going for walks, can help you build your relational skills.

An eating plan therapy is important to provide the necessary nutrients for your neurochemical needs.

You tend to have a problem staying with plans you make. Many life-style changes appear to oppose your neurochemical need. *You may be doing what others want, not what you need.* To continue on the road to recovery, you need to develop behavioral changes that are right for your brain, as described in this book.

TYPE C NEUROCHEMICAL PROFILE

If you have a Type C neurochemical profile, you probably have had long-term emotional or physical conflicts that create problems. Resolving guilt and encouraging forgiveness may help you. You can benefit from learning techniques that decrease your stress level.

Your neurochemical profile suggests that you show signs of behavioral compensation that aren't consistent with your reward center. Generally, you do things to try to feel better, but you may do them because of guilt or because others ask you to.

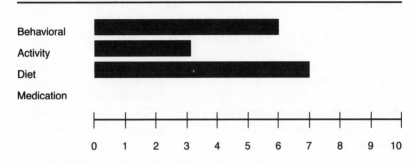

FIGURE 11-3
Recovery Effectiveness Rating

TYPE C PROFILE

It is better for you to engage in activities that satisfy your reward center and help your neurochemical imbalances.

Without resolving your spiritual conflicts, you are likely to transfer to another addiction or compulsion. I encourage you to confront issues and not avoid them.

You need to make behavioral changes to obtain rewards consistent with your neurochemical needs. You also may respond better to discussing problems with another individual rather than with a group. Activities with a group of people can be good if you are accepting of them and not judgmental.

You have a strong need to belong to groups, but the discussion could hinder your motivation to change. Don't be tempted to avoid change just because people understand you. Since you need support in relationship, you are particularly vulnerable to transferring to codependency or relationship addictions.

You do best in social situations that remain small, self-reflective, and supportive. Meditation, Bible studies, self-help, and emotionally supportive activities are probably most desirable. Marriage-enrichment or relationship-oriented activities can provide much help.

You can move into spirituality most effectively in churches with an emotional atmosphere and Bible study programs. If negative religious issues exist, consult the minister for help in developing intimacy in relationships.

Activity therapy is beneficial for health, but you'll probably be more open to accept it as a hobby or in quiet settings.

An eating plan therapy can be most beneficial, and with your Type C profile, you are likely to follow it closely.

TYPE D NEUROCHEMICAL PROFILE

If you have a Type D neurochemical profile, you probably have a genetic predisposition toward a depressed neurotransmission. Your family history may reveal alcoholism, depressive disorders, and compulsive or dysfunctional family systems. Your neurochemical profile describes genetic neurotransmitter alterations that hamper your ability to obtain rewards. You appear to do activities or behavior to treat the chemical imbalances in your brain consistent with your reward center. Essentially, your behavioral addiction is a "self-medication" of your neurochemical abnormality. Treatment of the neurochemical abnormality is essential to treat the behavioral issues.

Behavioral changes are essential to obtain rewards and remain consistent with neurochemical needs. Behavioral changes without medical or pharmacological intervention will not be as effective as behavioral changes with medication.

Group discussions in Bible studies or therapy sessions may be more acceptable to you than one-on-one conversation. You will be more comfortable in groups that allow independence;

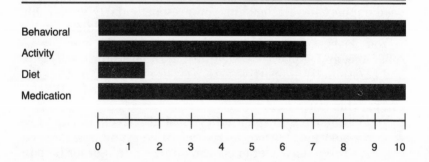

FIGURE 11-4
Recovery Effectiveness Rating

TYPE D PROFILE

dogmatic or critical groups make you uncomfortable. I encourage self-help fellowships. Become active in a church group. Recovery that deals with dysfunctional family systems may be important.

You will find social situations that include action or directed activities with some degree of structure more comfortable than other types of social settings. Intellectually or educationally oriented social activities can provide support.

Spirituality is most comfortable for you within a structured environment that does not have a strong emotional appeal. I recommend churches that emphasize teaching and study groups.

For emotional, neurochemical, and physical needs, I suggest activity and exercise therapy. You need activities that are healthy and relational. Doing activities with the family, spouse, or children may be very supportive.

An eating plan therapy is probably not as essential as in other profiles. However, a healthy diet is a good idea for everyone.

You may need medication and a medical evaluation for neurochemical manipulation. If you do need medication, talk with your physician and consider the following guidelines:

1. You have already changed your neurochemicals with alternative methods.

2. You now understand your specific goals for the use and effectiveness of medication.

3. You use specific alternative methods to reduce the amount of your medication as soon as possible.

4. You probably need medication if life-threatening situations exist, such as suicidal tendencies or severe depressions. After you have stabilized, your physician may help you develop goals for discontinuing or reevaluating the use of medication.

5. You should ask your physician to help you set goals so that you can eventually discontinue the medication.

6. You should not compromise your recovery by allowing such things as clinical depression or manic-depressive illness. The proper use of medication could enhance your recovery and reduce the chances for a relapse.

7. The use of mood-altering pharmaceuticals is rarely indicated in any disease in which a chemical dependency condition coexists.

TYPE E NEUROCHEMICAL PROFILE

If you have a Type E neurochemical profile, you probably show a genetic predisposition to enhanced neurotransmission. The family history may reveal alcoholism, anxiety disorders, or other compulsive or dysfunctional family systems. Your neurochemical profile describes genetic neurotransmitter alterations that hamper the ability to obtain rewards.

You appear to do activities or behavior to treat the chemical imbalances in your brain consistent with your reward center. Your behavioral addiction is possibly a "self-medication" of the neurochemical abnormality. Treatment of the neurochemical abnormality is necessary to treat your behavioral issues.

FIGURE 11-5
Recovery Effectiveness Rating

TYPE E PROFILE

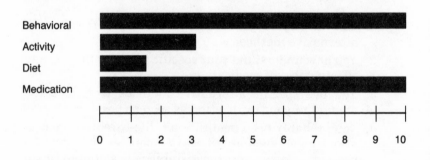

Behavioral changes are essential for you to obtain rewards and remain consistent with your neurochemical needs. Behavioral changes with the temporary use of medication may be more effective than behavioral changes alone. Discussing your problems with an individual may be more helpful than working with groups.

You will likely find help in group fellowship or churches

that focus on acceptance and belonging. The need to belong is vital, but the discussion in a group could lessen or eliminate your motivation to change. The transfer to codependency or relationship addiction is high. You also could benefit from pursuing your dysfunctional family issues.

Small social situations with an emphasis on self-reflection and support are effective. Meditation, Bible studies, self-help, and emotionally supportive activities are probably most desirable. Marriage-enrichment or relationship-oriented activities are important.

Churches that offer discussion-type settings can generally meet your spiritual needs. If you have unresolved negative religious issues, discuss them with a minister.

Activity therapy is beneficial for health but will probably be most acceptable through a hobby or in a quiet setting.

An eating plan therapy is probably not essential; however, a healthy diet is beneficial to anyone for maximum physical health.

A physician should help you decide whether to use medication. If the physician prescribes medicine, consider the following guidelines:

1. Remember that you tried to alter your neurochemical levels with alternative methods.
2. Before you start, set specific goals for the use of medication.
3. Use specific alternative methods to reduce your medication as soon as possible.
4. Set goals to discontinue medication in consultation with your physician.
5. If you have a life-threatening situation such as suicidal tendencies or severe depression, consult your physician and be ready to take medication. After you have stabilized, the physician may help you develop goals to discontinue medication or help to reevaluate your use of medication.
6. Don't compromise your recovery because of problems such as clinical depression or manic-depressive illness when the proper use of medication could enhance your recovery or at least reduce the possibility of relapse.

7. The use of mood-altering pharmaceuticals is rarely indicated in any disease in which a chemical dependency condition coexists.

TYPE F NEUROCHEMICAL PROFILE

If you have a Type F neurochemical profile, you are similar to persons who have been involved in long-term physical, spiritual, or emotional conflicts. You need encouragement to resolve your feelings of guilt and to forgive others. Learning techniques to decrease your level of stress may help.

You appear to do activities or behavior to treat the chemical imbalances in your brain not consistent with your reward center. You do better at activities to try to feel better. Do not, however, act because of guilt or because others urge you to. You need the type of activities that satisfy your reward center and balance your neurochemicals.

Without spiritual conflict resolution, you are likely to transfer to another addiction or compulsion. You also need to be encouraged not to avoid issues.

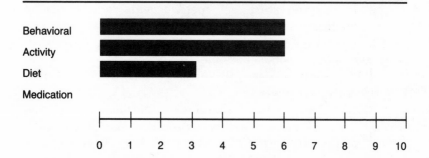

FIGURE 11-6
Recovery Effectiveness Rating

TYPE F PROFILE

Behavioral changes are important to obtain rewards and remain consistent with neurochemical needs. Behavioral changes without any consistent activity/exercise program will be less effective for you than if you use an activity/exercise program.

Group support and participation in church activities may be more effective than individual discussions with your support system. The group would be more effective if it has a purpose and direction. I encourage you to try self-help fellowships and active church involvement. You need support in building relationships. A strong temptation for you is to transfer to codependent or relationship addiction.

Social situations should include action/goal-directed activities with some degree of structure. Intellectually or educationally oriented social activities may be effective.

Your spiritual needs are best met in a teaching, structured environment that doesn't require you to participate through sharing unless you wish to. I recommend a church that emphasizes teaching and study groups.

Activity and exercise therapy is essential to meet your emotional and neurochemical and physical needs. Rewarding and relational activities are vital for you.

A healthy eating plan is suggested to provide the necessary proteins and amino acids for neurochemical demands.

TYPE G NEUROCHEMICAL PROFILE

If you have a Type G neurochemical profile, you probably have used drugs, alcohol, and/or medication or performed a compulsive behavior for a long period. Your profile is similar to that of persons whose neurochemistry has adapted to the consistent excitation of neurotransmitters by environmental, generational, or outside forces, such as diet, drugs, or consistent, long-term behavioral changes. Your enzymatic system may have adapted to such change.

It appears that the chemical changes in your brain are causing your behavior. Rewards for the behavior seem low. Transfer of addiction or compulsion may be low if you monitor your life-style and make changes.

Behavioral changes are important to obtain rewards and remain consistent with your neurochemical needs. Support from an individual is more readily accepted and effective than from groups. Group fellowships or church activities that focus on acceptance and belonging could be beneficial. The need to belong is essential, but the discussion in groups could eliminate your motivation to change.

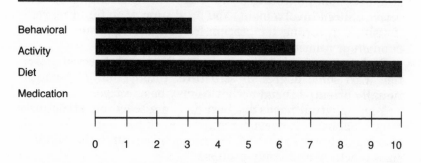

FIGURE 11-7
Recovery Effectiveness Rating

TYPE G PROFILE

I suggest you try social situations that remain small, self-reflective, and supportive. Meditation, Bible studies, self-help, and emotionally supportive activities are probably most desirable for you.

Your spiritual needs are best met in a teaching format that allows discussion. I recommend a church that emphasizes Bible study.

Activity therapy is beneficial for your health, but you will probably find it most acceptable in the form of a hobby or in a quiet setting.

An eating plan therapy can be most beneficial. You are more likely to follow an eating program than an activity program.

You tend to have problems with following your plan for any length of time. *You may be doing what others want you to do, not what is best for you.* You need to develop behavioral changes that are right for your brain, as I have described in this book.

TYPE H NEUROCHEMICAL PROFILE

If you have a Type H neurochemical profile, you probably show long-term genetic predispositions to compulsive disorders. Your family history may reveal alcoholism, perfectionism, compulsive overeating, or other compulsive disorders.

Your neurochemical profile indicates that neurochemical baseline levels or enzymatic levels that your brain considers normal are greater than those most people consider normal to have good feelings. That places you in an acceleration type of behavioral need; you constantly search for excitement.

There appears to be no behavioral compensation for such altered neurochemistry, which indicates you are responding to neurochemical abnormality. This situation can predispose you to transferring to another compulsion or addiction. Perhaps your goal in recovery should be to transfer to a positive addiction during the initial phase. Eliminating or minimizing compulsive behavior may be very difficult at first.

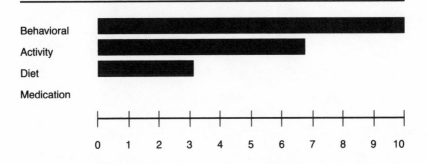

Figure 11-8
Recovery Effectiveness Rating

TYPE H PROFILE

Behavioral changes are essential for you to obtain rewards and remain consistent with your neurochemical needs. Behavioral changes without any consistent activity/exercise program will be less than with the activity/exercise program. Group systems and activities may be more effective support systems than individual interaction. I strongly encourage attendance at self-help fellowships or active church participation.

Social situations should include action/goal-directed activities with some degree of structure. Intellectually or educationally oriented social activities may be most acceptable to you.

Spiritual needs can be met effectively through a high-energy, intellectually stimulating environment that doesn't require you to participate through sharing groups unless you want to. I recommend a church that emphasizes teaching and study groups.

Activity and exercise therapy is essential for your emotional and neurochemical needs and your physical health. Relational high-energy activities are necessary for you to improve your self-esteem and to strengthen relationships.

An eating plan therapy provides the necessary protein and amino acid substances that form the neurochemicals your body needs. You may resist dietary issues and be noncompliant if you don't work hard at it.

You may tend to have a problem following through with your actions because you like to move from one activity or plan to another without completing any of them. I urge you to focus on one activity at a time. If your recovery is to be successful, you need to work at being more self-disciplined.

12

— ♥ —

Balancing Act

"I don't know much about dieting," Susan said, "except, of course, not to eat carbohydrates." She patted her thighs. "That's where they end up."

"I thought it was high carbohydrates and low fats," said Skip, her husband. "Or was it high protein and low carbohydrates?"

Their confusion isn't unusual. For the past twenty years, self-styled dietitians and weight-loss experts set up rules that they didn't fully understand themselves.

Here is one thing you do need to know: Your body has to have carbohydrates—a major percentage of your total food intake! In this chapter, I want to help you understand what it means to balance your diet with carbohydrates, proteins, and fats.

♥ ♥ ♥

Amino acids are the foundation of any sensible eating plan. Protein is made up of amino acids. You get protein from meat, poultry, fish, and animal products such as milk and cheese.

Several amino acids tie together to make protein, so there are various names for amino acids. Phenylalanine, tyrosine, leucine, isoleucine, valine, isovaline, and others make up the whole nature of protein.

Even though you find amino acids in various products, fish have a different amino acid makeup from that of turkey, which is different from that of beef, which is different from that of pork products. In your choice of an eating plan you'll need to look at which amino acids you want to use. I'll help you see which ones are preferable for you while you also seek the minimal amount of fat.

Why amino acids? Your body has to convert or break down protein into amino acids. Then the amino acids are broken down so they can be transmitted through the bloodstream to the brain.

Certain neurotransmitters require specific amino acids. For example, tyrosine is an amino acid found in red meats. Within minutes after you eat, your body breaks down the food, and the amino acids in the meat are converted to a neurochemical called norepinephrine. You immediately feel an inflow of energy. If you need more energy or suffer from depression, norepinephrine is a natural, safe way to alleviate those symptoms. However, you can't take neurotransmitters—only the amino acids.

Tyrosine also converts into dopamine. If your dopamine level is too high, you may experience stress-related reality disturbances, fears, and paranoia. In fact, schizophrenics have too high a level of dopamine. If it is too low, depression can occur. As you can imagine, balancing the amount of dopamine is essential. Dopamine and norepinephrine are related and are called adrenergic neurotransmitters.

Another amino acid, tryptophan, converts to serotonin. That is the more quieting, more focusing neurotransmitter. Persons deficient in serotonin may be scattered and depressed and have low energy.

If you have done your neurochemical evaluation, you are now aware of your neurotransmission levels. It is beyond the scope of a book to define your exact neurochemical levels, but we can give you guidelines. You can design your eating plan based upon symptoms we will discuss later. A neurochemical evaluation can give your physician more specific information and is available through the Robertson Institute. I will help you design your own eating plan based on those results, including how to increase or decrease your amino acids according to your need. If you are like most people, you can get all your needed amino acids in a natural form through food.

Typically, most people don't meet their needs naturally—through intelligent eating—for two reasons.

1. *You are pill dependent.* Think about the times when you used food to take away a bad feeling or to lessen it. If you were angry, if you felt rejected, or if you experienced some other emotional reactions, you might have turned to food. If you can relate to feeding yourself when you feel bad, your personality is such that you'll tend to grab a pill to cure your pain: aspirin for headaches, antacid for upset stomachs, and a laxative for constipation. You don't seek natural ways of curing these ailments. For you, pills are the natural way.

I urge you to concentrate on behavioral manipulation. It will help you find other ways to reduce your negative emotions instead of using a pill.

2. *You deplete your amino acids or neurotransmitters by overeating.* You will learn that a good, balanced eating plan can be extremely effective in bringing your amino acid level back to normal within a short period of time. When you eat a large amount of food, certain amino acids compete with other amino acids for absorption. For example, the larger amino acids such as leucine, valine, isovaline, and isoleucine will prevent tryptophan from being absorbed across the blood-brain barrier (or from getting to the brain). This could cause a depletion in serotonin levels, since they are manufactured from tryptophan. A symptom of serotonin deficiency can be depression and carbohydrate craving. Both will complicate diet recovery.

When you eat anything, the food immediately goes through the digestive process. The food is broken down and pushed into the bloodstream. From there, this converted form of "food" goes through the liver and is converted into different energy products, all of which are used by parts of your brain and body. For example, your pancreas makes and releases insulin. It also responds to hormonal effects from your brain that decide how much insulin to release into the blood and how much to store or absorb within the pancreas. This balance is affected, of course, by the way you eat.

Because of the way the conversion of food takes place in your body, one day of following the best eating plan in the world won't give you an adequate response. It takes several weeks of following your eating plan. Over the course of weeks, you may eat and feel almost immediate relief. Yet the next time, you feel no emotional or physical response. Don't be concerned. The key is consistency. Follow the eating plan. Over a period of time, your consistency does pay off—usually two weeks to six weeks. How long it takes for your body to respond regularly to the proper nutritional input will depend largely on how you treated your body before you started this style of eating.

WARNING: Please get a checkup first. Your body needs to be healthy or disease treated to be in diet therapy. Furthermore, certain diseases require diets different from those described. Please follow your physician's recommendations.

GENERAL EATING GUIDELINES

Before we get to your specific diet, let's look at general eating guidelines.

1. Please heed this warning. If your physician has suggested an alternative eating plan for medical or other conditions, please follow that advice. Diet can be used to control cholesterol, salt intake, high blood pressure, diabetes, and other already existing conditions.

2. If you have food allergies, please make alternative food choices in the same category.

3. If you have high blood pressure or suffer from hypertension, you probably know (and I remind you) that high-sodium foods are inappropriate for you. As you go through the eating plan, you may want to eliminate high-sodium foods.

4. As I've already stated, the goal of this eating plan is not weight reduction. Even though I sometimes use the word *diet*, it means a balanced arrangement of what you eat, the amount you eat, and the combinations of food. This then becomes a balanced and neurochemically oriented dietary arrangement. *It is an eating plan for your emotions*.

5. The body needs carbohydrates to function. However, to many people, carbohydrates (which are found in starches such as potatoes and simple sugars) mean weight gain.

"I always thought that if I just cut down my carbo intake to the minimum, I'd lose weight and keep it off," said Angela.

Unfortunately, she missed the whole point. Persons who

eliminate carbohydrates necessarily limit their eating plan to protein and some fat, which is not healthy eating.

"Angela," I said, "your body does need carbohydrates to function properly. Carbohydrates provide energy precursors. That means you need carbohydrates to make tryptophan and other chemicals and hormones necessary for brain chemistry regulation."

I also explained the difference between simple and complex carbohydrates. "You really need *complex* carbohydrates because they are released more slowly and more effectively than simple sugars." I explained that eating simple carbohydrates such as cake or any sweet-tasting food is like trying to keep a fire going with kindling—small, thin sticks of wood. You can get a quick amount of heat, but it burns up rapidly. Getting complex carbohydrates to burn takes a little longer, but they burn over a longer period. Or you can think of simple carbohydrates as fast-burning fuel in a gas tank. You get high speed for a short distance. You have to continue adding more and more of this fuel to keep the energy level going. By contrast, complex carbohydrates burn more slowly and evenly and give you a smoother ride.

6. Eating three meals a day is better than skipping meals. A lot of people tend to skip meals:

- They get too busy so they "just snack a little here and there." (They usually eat more than a normal meal that way.)
- They think they can lose weight. (This method almost never works. They more than make up on the meals they actually do eat.)
- They think of food as their enemy and their downfall. (You need food for survival, energy, and emotional balance.)

You set yourself up for problems if you start playing with your hormonal system by skipping meals. For example, if you eat a heavy meal of carbohydrates from simple sugars such as doughnuts or pancakes in the morning, you produce a lot of insulin. It is trying to pull in the glucose that has been converted from carbohydrates. You get a big rush of energy—for a period of time. If you don't eat for eight hours, your blood sugar level drops, but the insulin is too high because it takes time for it to go down. If you don't eat then, you feel tired, moody, and maybe depressed. To avoid this, you need to learn to stay within a consistent eating plan that has more complex carbohydrates.

7. Balance each meal with proteins and fats. A balance doesn't mean fifty-fifty, however. A small percentage of your eating plan can be fats. Most Americans make fats more than 30 percent of their diet, which is far too much for good health. Balance depends on whether you are reducing, but it may be in the following ranges:

proteins	15 to 25 percent
carbohydrates	50 to 60 percent
fats	20 to 30 percent

An eating plan too high in fat content can result in arteriosclerosis and cardiac problems. An overload of simple and/or complex carbohydrates can cause mood swings and vitamin deficiencies. Consuming too much protein can lead to liver and kidney problems.

─────────── ♥ ♥ ♥ ───────────

Balance is the key.

♥ ♥ ♥

───────────

8. Avoid alcohol. Whether you're an alcoholic or a social drinker, alcohol plays havoc

- with your mind from the physiological standpoint.
- with your health from a medical standpoint.
- with your emotions and attitudes from a spiritual standpoint.

At this point of your food-recovery program, it's essential for you to stop drinking alcohol so that your brain can function normally.

9. Eliminate or limit caffeine. For some people, one or two cups of coffee each day may not be a problem. For others, any caffeine interferes with their health. If you drink more than

six cups of coffee a day, you really need to limit your caffeine intake. Caffeine is contained in many products including tea, chocolate, some aspirin-type products, and soft drinks. By checking labels you can see which are caffeine free and which contain caffeine.

10. Trim all visible fat from your meat. Take the skin off turkey and chicken because it is almost totally composed of fat. Cutting your fat consumption may be difficult because fat gives flavor to your food. But you can cut the amount drastically, still enjoy good taste, and, most of all, benefit from lower cholesterol levels.

11. Replace saturated fats with polyunsaturated fats and decrease the amount of fats. Polyunsaturated fats are usable fats, whereas saturated fats can increase your cholesterol level. Most animal fats are saturated fats, while vegetable fats have higher polyunsaturated fats. Vegetable fats are found in corn oil, cottonseed oil, margarine, and other vegetable oils.

12. Decrease your consumption of high-cholesterol foods, such as butter, cheese, and other dairy products. For most people, I suggest cutting down the number of eggs consumed. That means no more than two or three eggs a week in any form, including baked goods. However, the elderly, children, and premenopausal women sometimes benefit from eating eggs.

I urge you to eliminate or drastically reduce these high-cholesterol sources

- if cholesterol has ever been a problem.
- if you are male.
- if you are postmenopausal.

These are the three high-risk categories for high cholesterol.

13. Decrease your consumption of processed and refined sugars, such as sodas, cereal, and the sugar you add to cereal and coffee.

14. Decrease your consumption of salt and foods high in salt content.

15. Whenever possible, use fresh foods instead of processed foods because they have a higher vitamin content.

16. Avoid frying or immersing foods in fat, such as French fries or taco chips. Learn to eat food that is broiled, steamed, or

baked. These three processes help foods maintain their vitamin and mineral content.

You'll learn about your specific eating plan in the next chapter.

♥ ♥ ♥

Vital facts about myself: I commit myself to a balanced eating plan because it will benefit me. I commit myself to learn to use this balanced eating plan the rest of my life.

♥ ♥ ♥

13

♥

Eating Right

A healthy eating plan for you

- follows general guidelines.
- speeds along your recovery.
- follows your neurochemical profile.
- helps to alter your neurochemical baseline levels.
- improves your moods and emotions temporarily.

If you are a Type A, B, C, or D profile and you follow the eating plan for a Type E, F, G, or H profile, you will become more depressed and function with less clarity. The eating plan recommended to you is to increase your neurotransmission and increase focus or concentration.

I have divided the eating plan types into two categories: (1) eating plans that *enhance* neurotransmission, and (2) eating plans that *inhibit* neurotransmission. Your moods, clarity of thinking, and energy levels are affected by neurotransmission levels. These levels may be altered by the level of amino acids in the brain. These levels are affected by the foods you eat and the manner in which you eat them.

If you are neurochemical profile Type A, B, C, or D, you will benefit from eating plans that improve neurotransmission. (Types A and C usually follow eating plans better than Types B and D.)

If you are neurochemical profile Type E, F, G, or H, you will benefit from eating plans that inhibit neurotransmission.

(Types E and G are usually willing to follow eating plans, but Types F and H tend to resist.)

To be workable, an eating program must take into consideration medical complications. If you suffer from heart disease, diabetes, or other conditions that require a special diet, you would be wise to follow your physician-prescribed eating plan unless your physician approves the following eating plan.

EATING PLAN TO IMPROVE NEUROTRANSMISSION

The adrenergic-rich eating plan enhances neurotransmission. Neurochemical profile Types A, B, C, and D can begin with this diet. The eating plan will help you decrease depression. Because of the complex nature of neurochemistry, you should review your symptoms to develop a plan geared more for your needs.

The adrenergic-rich eating plan is a high protein and complex carbohydrate diet.

The recommended high protein foods are listed in order of preference: fish, chicken (no skin), veal, lean trimmed beef, low fat milk products, soybeans, whole milk, cold cuts, pork and pork products (lean or low fat preferred), and lamb.

The recommended complex carbohydrate portion of the plan is as follows: vegetables—beans, beets, broccoli, carrots, corn, cucumbers, lettuce, mushrooms, and squash; fresh fruits—apples, bananas, berries, grapes, grapefruit, kiwifruit, mangoes, melons, pears, and fruit juices (no sugar added); grains/starches—brown rice, whole grain breads, pasta, bagels, potatoes, and crackers.

Those following the adrenergic-rich eating plan generally should avoid snacking on the following grains and starches: breads, crackers, muffins, rolls, bagels, pasta, potatoes, rice, corn, and barley.

EATING PLAN TO DECREASE NEUROTRANSMISSION

The tryptophan-rich eating plan decreases neurotransmission. Neurochemical profile Types E, F, G, and H can begin with this plan and adapt it to fit individual symptoms.

The tryptophan-rich eating plan is a modified high protein and complex carbohydrate diet.

The recommended modified high protein portion of the plan includes the following: fish, turkey, and milk products (low fat).

The recommended complex carbohydrate portion of the plan is as follows: vegetables—beans, beets, broccoli, carrots, corn, cucumbers, lettuce, mushrooms, and squash; fresh fruits—apples, bananas, berries, grapes, grapefruit, kiwifruit, mangoes, melons, pears, and fruit juices (no sugar added); grains/starches—brown rice, whole grain breads, pasta, bagels, potatoes, and crackers.

Those following the tryptophan-rich eating plan should avoid or use sparingly the following: beef, cold cuts (unless low fat), pork and pork products, and lamb.

Those following the tryptophan-rich eating plan should totally avoid the following: coffee, chocolate, and other products containing caffeine.

LIST OF SYMPTOMS

The purpose of this symptoms list is to help you with any special emotional issues you have by using food. Instead of self-medicating and exacerbating your condition, you can use food as an ally.

Although I can show you the type of foods to eat, bear these facts in mind:

1. Using such foods for particular needs is no guaranteed cure. What I suggest does work for most people.
2. Permission to eat is not permission to eat an unlimited amount. I suggest you eat only normal portions.
3. For any suggested foods, you will need to eat them regularly for a period up to six weeks before you become aware of a distinct improvement.
4. You are committing yourself to follow these eating plans indefinitely. These eating plans are not intended to be a restrictive diet that you follow only until you reach a particular weight. Your aim is to make lifelong changes in your eating patterns.

I'm including a list of symptoms and diet considerations to help in establishing an eating plan to fit your needs. The symptoms listed below are those that are not frequently influenced by outside factors, such as medical condition, grief over death of a loved one, or loss of a job.

Follow these eating plans daily.

SYMPTOMS	FOOD PLAN
Anxiety	Tryptophan-rich plan
Depression	Either plan or both
Difficulty focusing or concentrating	Tryptophan-rich plan
Anger	Adrenergic-rich plan
Difficulty sleeping	Tryptophan-rich plan
Lack of energy and motivation	Adrenergic-rich plan
Craving carbohydrates	Tryptophan-rich plan

COMBINING EATING PLANS

You may need both eating plans. As laid out, they do interfere with each other, but you can make adjustments and successfully combine them.

Here are some guidelines to consider when combining eating plans:

1. Use the adrenergic-rich eating plan during the day when the tyrosine and phenylalanine are absorbed.

2. Don't eat high-protein foods after six o'clock in the evening since they will interfere with tryptophan absorption.

3. A small amount of food rich in complex carbohydrates and tryptophan makes an appropriate snack at night.

If you take the adrenergic-rich eating plan early enough, there will be no problem with the tryptophan at night. Of course, you need to decrease your caloric intake if you add the nighttime snack.

MOODS AND FOODS

You may go through various periods in a single day or week when outside influences create stress or depression. These are temporary and normal. For example, if someone close to you gets injured, you will probably be stressed. As the worry over that person's life is relieved, your stress level drops. That is a natural response. If you are depressed or stressed without outside influences, your baseline neurotransmission levels are out of balance.

Changing your style of eating naturally affects your feelings. Such mood swings are typical of the temporary neurochemical changes, and they are unrelated to your baseline level of neurotransmission. Your baseline level is the *overall* feeling of depression or anxiety you experience with no interference from outside influences.

FOODS TO INCREASE CONCENTRATION

Often the release of excitatory neurochemicals can cause you to have scattered thoughts. Your thoughts may not seem logical or consistent. Or you have a problem completing tasks. This reaction is normal. The overstimulation of your nervous system causes the multiple firing of nerves. You then have difficulty concentrating.

Manipulating or changing eating patterns has proven helpful to many persons who have an occasional lack of concentration. Tryptophan can help in concentration. A turkey sandwich, low-fat milk products, and cheese improve concentration by providing a temporary feedback to the adrenergic system.

Concentration can also be affected by depression or other psychological or medical disorders. If poor concentration continues, you may wish to have medical and neurochemical evaluations.

FOODS TO DECREASE ANXIETY

The release of excessive amounts of excitatory neurotransmitters causes anxiety. Exercise is usually the most effective method to "burn up" these neurotransmitters. However, a change in your eating plan can also be beneficial.

Cutting down on foods that directly stimulate you decreases temporary anxiety conditions. Avoiding red meat, caffeine, and chocolate usually helps. You may also respond to an increase in tryptophan during this time. Turkey, pasta, fish, and low-fat cheese decrease anxiety.

Psychological and medical conditions affect anxiety. If your anxiety persists, you should have medical and neurochemical evaluations done.

FOODS TO RELIEVE DEPRESSION

The type of depression helped by a healthy eating plan is the temporary "down feeling," not the overwhelming chronic type. Increasing the amount of excitatory neurochemicals improves mood. Cereals, fish, chicken, veal, and beef relieve depression. Eat a meal rich in protein and drink a cup of coffee to increase the amount of excitatory neurochemicals. If you feel you need to continue this program daily, I suggest further evaluation.

FOODS TO DECREASE STRESS

When you feel you are under stress, avoid coffee, chocolate, and red meat. Since stress causes a release of excitatory neurotransmitters, you don't need more stimulation. Vegetables, fresh fruits, salads, breads, and pasta decrease stress.

Stress is emotionally, physically, and spiritually destructive. The medical and emotional consequences of stress vary from high blood pressure to anxiety or depression. Handling stress as quickly as possible is important. Temporary relief of the neurochemical alterations prevents or minimizes the medical and psychological consequences.

AMINO ACID SUPPLEMENTS

Amino acid supplements won't significantly affect baseline neurotransmitters unless you have a dietary or drug-induced deficiency. However, they can have considerable direct effects on your moods.

If tyrosine is taken one hour before meals, the stimulating effect can decrease the appetite. Any genetic or baseline neurotransmitter alteration overrides this effect. Compulsive overeating requires balancing the baseline neurotransmitters for appetite suppression to occur.

Phenylalanine comes in d and l derivatives. The d is for persons who experience chronic pain. Taken by itself, d phenylalanine may not provide much of an effect; however, when it is combined with certain anti-inflammatory agents and analgesics, it may prove beneficial.

If you need an adrenergic-rich eating plan and are underweight, you may prefer l phenylalanine. Tyrosine can affect your weight even though it lessens your depression.

Please remember this: A healthy eating plan is essential for the brain to change. Otherwise, the brain may want to change, but it won't have the necessary nutrients.

♥ ♥ ♥

A vital fact about myself: Because I want to change, I follow a sensible and healthy eating plan.

♥ ♥ ♥

14

— ♥ —

Exercising for a Healthy Brain

Exercise directly affects your brain. Through exercise, you can increase or decrease your neurochemicals. The proper use of exercise and physical activity can play a significant role in your recovery process. The type of activity you do regularly will affect your reward center and your neurochemical baseline. Consequently, I believe in prescribing activities in the same way medicine is prescribed. Just as you follow your eating plan, by using exercise and activities, you can receive direct, although temporary, results.

EXERCISE AND NEUROTRANSMISSION

I urge exercise for two reasons: (1) Activity increases or decreases your neurochemicals and helps to alter your baseline neurochemical levels, and (2) if you feel better, you look better, and you are healthier.

The benefit of your exercise program depends on your medical condition. If you have any physical restrictions, please follow your physician's guidelines. You can use other methods to change your neurochemistry.

I like to combine a healthy eating plan with an effective exercise program. Through running, weight lifting, racquetball, basketball, and other forms of physical movement, you stimulate your cardiovascular system. In the activities list, I call these Type E (for excitatory) activities. By contrast, Type I (for inhibitory) activities are less strenuous but require more concentration (and less cardiovascular involvement). Such activities include playing card games, watching quiet movies, woodworking, and doing other hobbies.

At first, cardiovascular exercise (or Type E activities) burns up excitatory neurochemicals. If the activities are done daily for thirty to forty-five days, they release endorphins. This reward neurochemical is the one that causes the *runner's high,* a term popularized by long-distance runners who speak of a feeling of peace or a sense of well-being.

Cardiovascular exercise affects brain chemistry. If you exercise daily for at least two months, you will most likely develop an increase in neurotransmission. Running two to three days a week, with a break on alternate days, burns up excitatory neurotransmitters without causing runner's high. Following a moderate exercise program would decrease neurotransmission by burning up neurochemicals.

However, you may be one of those individuals who just doesn't get a reward from cardiovascular exercise or Type E activities. You may respond better to a prescribed eating plan or Type I activities. Type I activities can alter your neurotransmitters by focusing the thoughts and energy. The relaxing and focusing increase certain neurochemicals. Properly prescribing these activities can enhance or decrease neurotransmission levels.

EXERCISE/ACTIVITY AND NEUROCHEMICAL PROFILES

To set up your own exercise and activity program, fill out an activities list. Refer to your neurochemical profile to help you select your activity program.

Daily routine exercise plans affect neurochemical baseline levels. Alleviation-of-stress activities are used when persons feel out of balance so they can temporarily relieve their neurochemical imbalances.

ACTIVITIES LIST

Complete the activities list to help you decide on the activities and hobbies you most enjoy. You can also substitute activities that require the same amount of effort.

Each of the activities has an *I* (or inhibitory) or *E* (or excitatory) effect. These are the general effects. You may find a particular activity listed as *I* is actually excitatory to you. If that is the case, consider it to be an *E* activity. The same is true if an *E* activity is actually an *I* to you.

Check the activities you have participated in and enjoyed.

Outdoors
- ☐ Boating (E)
- ☐ Camping (I)
- ☐ Fishing (I)
- ☐ Hiking (I)
- ☐ Hunting (I)
- ☐ Other:
  _____
  _____

Family
- ☐ Get-togethers (I)
- ☐ Picnics (I)
- ☐ Trips/travel (I)
- ☐ Walks (I)
- ☐ Other:
  _____
  _____

Church
- ☐ Bible study (I)
- ☐ Church services (I, E)
- ☐ Get-togethers (I)
- ☐ Teach or attend Sunday school (I)
- ☐ Other:
  _____
  _____

> Key:
> E = Excitatory
> I = Inhibitory

Sports
- ☐ Aerobics (I, E)
- ☐ Biking (E)
- ☐ Dancing (E)
- ☐ Fitness class (E)
- ☐ Golf (E)
- ☐ Jogging (E)
- ☐ Paddleball (E)
- ☐ Racquetball (E)
- ☐ Skiing (E)
- ☐ Swimming (E)
- ☐ Team sports:
  _____
- ☐ Tennis (E)
- ☐ Walking (I)
- ☐ Weight lifting (E)
- ☐ Other:
  _____
  _____

Motor Sports
- ☐ ATV (E)
- ☐ Dirt bike (E)
- ☐ Four-wheel/off-road driving (E)
- ☐ Motorcycle (road) (E)
- ☐ Snowmobile (E)
- ☐ Vintage/classic cars (I, E)
- ☐ Other:
  _____
  _____

Nonphysical (Hobbies)
- ☐ Attend sporting events (I):
  _____
  _____
- ☐ Billiards (I)
- ☐ Cards (I)
- ☐ Carpentry (I)
- ☐ Collect things (I)
- ☐ Computers (I)
- ☐ Crafts (I):
  _____
- ☐ Creative writing (I)
- ☐ Go to movies/ plays/concerts (I)
- ☐ Landscaping (I)
- ☐ Music
  - ☐ Play (E)
  - ☐ Listen (I)
- ☐ Painting (art) (I)
- ☐ Puzzles
  - ☐ Crosswords (I)
  - ☐ Jigsaw (I)
- ☐ Reading (I)
- ☐ Table games (I)
- ☐ Video games (I)
- ☐ Watch TV (I)
- ☐ Woodworking (I)
- ☐ Work on cars (I)
- ☐ Other:
  _____
  _____

ACTIVITY PROGRAM FOR TYPE A AND TYPE C PROFILES

If you have a Type A or C profile, your goal is to increase certain neurochemical levels through activities. Exercise can be of some help for Type A or C individuals.

Develop an exercise program that consists of *I* activities from the activities list.

Do a five-minute warm-up, such as walking or stretching.

Do a twenty-minute exercise from the *I* list.

Do a five-minute cool down, such as walking or stretching.

—Schedule—

	Sun	Mon	Tue	Wed	Thur	Fri	Sat
Routine	I	I	I	I	I	I	I

To relieve stress, perform *E* activities.

Routine *I* Activities (used to change baseline levels)

_____

_____

_____

Stress-Relief *E* Activities (used to feel better temporarily)

_____

_____

Follow the routine schedule to keep in balance. When you feel out of balance, uptight, or anxious, stress-relief activities will alleviate the pressure.

ACTIVITY PROGRAM FOR TYPE F AND TYPE H PROFILES

If you have a Type F or H profile, you will benefit at least moderately from an exercise program. The goal is to burn up excitatory neurotransmitters, causing a decrease in neurochemical baseline levels.

Develop an exercise program consisting of routine *E* activities alternating with routine *I* activities. Select *I* and *E* activities from the activities list.

Do a five-minute warm-up, such as walking or stretching.

Do a twenty-minute exercise from the *I* list alternating with activities from the *E* list.

Do a five-minute cool down, such as walking or stretching.

—Schedule—

	Sun	Mon	Tue	Wed	Thur	Fri	Sat
Routine	I	E	I	E	I	E	I

To relieve stress, perform *E* or additional activities.

Routine *E* Activities   Routine *I* Activities

_____   _____

_____   _____

Stress-Relief *E* Activities

_____

_____

Follow the routine schedule to keep in balance. When you feel out of balance, uptight, or depressed, stress-relief activities will alleviate the pressure.

ACTIVITY PROGRAM FOR TYPE E AND TYPE G PROFILES

If you have a Type E profile, you receive some benefit from the exercise program, but if you are Type G, you receive moderate to high benefits. Feedback systems are used to decrease neurotransmission levels.

Develop an exercise program that consists of *I* activities from the activities list.

Do a five-minute warm-up, such as walking or stretching.

Do a twenty-minute exercise from the *I* list.

Do a five-minute cool down, such as walking or stretching.

—Schedule—

	Sun	Mon	Tue	Wed	Thur	Fri	Sat
Routine	I		I		I		I

To relieve stress, perform *I* or additional activities.

Routine *I* Activities (used to change baseline levels)

_____

_____

Stress-Relief *I* Activities (used to feel better temporarily)

_____

_____

Follow the routine schedule to keep in balance. When you feel out of balance, uptight, or depressed, stress-relief activities will alleviate the pressure.

ACTIVITY PROGRAM FOR TYPE B AND TYPE D PROFILES

If you have a Type B profile, you will benefit greatly from your activity program. It is an essential part of your recovery.

If you are Type D, you will benefit moderately from your exercise program. You will use indirect methods to enhance neurotransmission, which results in the runner's high. Even though the exercise program may feel uncomfortable for the first thirty to forty-five days, you will start to feel better. You may need to exert self-discipline in combination with an adrenergic-rich food program for the first two months.

Develop an exercise program that consists of routine *E* activities from the activities list.

Do a five-minute warm-up, such as walking or stretching.

Do a twenty-minute exercise from the *E* list.

Do a five-minute cool down, such as walking or stretching.

—Schedule—

	Sun	Mon	Tue	Wed	Thur	Fri	Sat
Routine	E	E	E	E	E	E	E

To relieve stress, perform *E* or additional activities.

Routine *E* Activities (used to change baseline levels)

_____

_____

Stress-Relief *E* Activities (used to feel better temporarily)

_____

_____

Follow the routine schedule to keep in balance. When you feel out of balance, uptight, or depressed, stress-relief activities will alleviate the pressure.

The exercise programs listed here are important to follow. They provide neurochemical changes and stress relief and balance. Although some persons resist and don't get much of a reward, I still encourage them to participate in some type of activity or hobby.

FIGURE 14-1
Activities Program

	TYPE OF NEUROCHEMICAL PROFILE							
	A	B	C	D	E	F	G	H
Activities to change baseline levels	I	E	I	E	I	I,E	I	I,E
Activities for temporary stress relief	E	E	E	E	I	E	I	E
Additional activities to relieve objective stress	E	E	E	E	E	E	E	E
Additional activities to relieve subjective stress	E/I	E/I	E/I	E/I	E/I	E/I	E/I	E/I

Key: E = Excitatory; I = Inhibitory

ACTIVITY GUIDELINES

1. The goal of an activity is not to make you more muscular or to help you perform better in any specific area. The goal is to promote your health and emotional well-being.

2. It is easier to follow a daily routine than a hit-or-miss approach.

3. If you begin to feel light-headed or uncomfortable while doing your activity, stop. Seek professional advice.

4. If you begin to have more physical or emotional complications after beginning to exercise, consult your physician.

5. Before beginning any exercise program, consult your physician to determine your activity.

ACTIVITY AND STRESS

These exercise programs affect baseline neurotransmitters. Follow them daily to get the maximum benefit.

Exercise relieves stress by changing neurotransmitters and also prevents stress through neurochemical baseline stabilization.

The type of activity you find to alleviate your stress is highly individualized. However, you should consider two different types of stressful situations.

1. Objective stress refers to stress from situations outside yourself—the kind you can't change, such as taxation, war, inflation, and often company policies. This type of stress creates a neurochemical release. To get relief, a Type *E* workout is generally more effective than Type *I* activities.

2. Subjective stress comes from within. It is that feeling you need to change, but you're afraid to change. Usually it's an unidentified stress and shows through a lack of energy or focus. The cause may be feelings of inadequacy, insecurity, and loneliness. Hobbies or fun activities of Type *I* or Type *E* may help you overcome this type of stress.

♥ ♥ ♥

Diet and activity programs begin to get the brain ready for behavioral and thought changes. It is essential that you follow these programs. Since change can be stressful, you must be in good physical health and have some knowledge of stress-relief techniques. Neurochemicals that are beginning to achieve a better balance also perceive behavioral changes more accurately.

Once you have begun the activity and eating plan programs, you can then work on behavioral and thought changes.

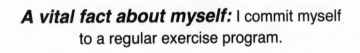

A *vital fact about myself:* I commit myself to a regular exercise program.

15

♥

Emotional Triggers

I had known William for years. Although an able speaker, he was no stand-up comedian like Jay Leno. One time he was invited to be the keynote speaker at a prestigious banquet honoring volunteers in the community. Because I was sitting only feet away from the speaker's table and facing him, I noticed what he ate and drank before he spoke. William drank two glasses of wine, turned down the vegetables, and ignored his green salad. He ate a meal heavy with starchy foods and finished with helpings of two rich desserts. That was unusual for William. He rarely drank even one glass of wine, and because of a heart condition, he tried to eat carefully balanced meals. Only a few weeks earlier he told me, "I eat sweets about six times in any given year."

That night, William spoke for nearly an hour. People laughed politely at his badly timed jokes and applauded courteously at the end. My wife and I felt a little sad for him.

A few days later, William and I ran into each other at the post office. The subject of the banquet came up. "You know, it was one of the best nights of my life," he said. "Every line just flowed. Every joke was perfect." He paused to say that he hadn't prepared well, had been scared he wouldn't do a good job, and was extremely nervous until he actually stood up to speak.

"And then the words flowed," he said. For a few minutes William glowed as he talked about his good form and how free he had felt that night. I don't recall what I said, but it was as little as possible.

What was going on? Along with his six or eight ounces of alcohol, William had a meal loaded with simple carbohydrates that went immediately into his bloodstream. The food and alcohol so altered his brain chemistry that William misperceived reality. His inflated sense of well-being made it seem that everything he said rang with wit.

William's food and alcohol intake had given him a false perception of who he was. In one sense, I could say that people didn't see the real William. They saw a man under the influence of chemicals, even though those were mostly food chemicals.

When William came to the banquet, already nervous and afraid that he wouldn't do a good job, two things happened that *triggered* something in his brain. First, he was undergoing emotional stress (he was nervous and afraid). Second, he was in a situation where he responded to his triggers. Had he been aware of the triggers, he could have taken preventive action. Unfortunately, William was unaware.

This situation isn't unusual. Many of us have hidden, self-destructive automatic responses to triggers. Unless we become aware of them, we get in trouble without knowing what's going on.

Many people work hard at their weight-loss programs. They lose the pounds they set up as goals. Then something happens. They blow the diet, and the weight creeps back on.

Too many diet programs aren't very good at helping their clients keep the weight off. The major reason, I'm convinced, is that the experts don't know about triggers.

Before I go further, I'd like to define my use of the term *triggers*. To do that, I again refer to the work of Ivan Pavlov. In his experiments, after the pattern had formed in the dogs' brains (bell = food), the dogs could do nothing but salivate upon hearing the bell. The bell became the trigger. Nothing happened until that sound filled the animals' ears.

Because of Pavlov's pioneer work, one of the things we've learned in the past eighty years is this: *Outside influences trigger physiological responses in the brain.* The canines salivated without having a logical reason to do so. The experiment was successful for one reason only: Over an extended period of time, the dogs had been drilled (programmed or brainwashed) to associate the ringing of the bell with the delivery of food.

From a practical viewpoint, what does this mean for you and your problems with food dependency? At some time in the past, quite likely in childhood, you were programmed to respond automatically. You didn't hear a bell, but something triggered an action. As soon as it happened, you immediately wanted food.

That trigger is an outside influence. It causes an internal conflict, which results in an automatic response in your brain. The response is probably hidden from your conscious thinking, but you can locate it. Right now, you're so used to your automatic response, you don't even hear the bell or realize that it sounded. You have an emotional and physiological response to your trigger—and you probably have more than one. You prepare to eat. You may not literally salivate, but you feel hungry, your stomach yearns for something to come inside, or your mind fills with thoughts of food. Any of these effects has come about because of your trigger.

Here's how you might have acquired your trigger. When you were a child, let's say you noticed something about your father's behavior. After he argued with your mother or lost his temper, he went to the refrigerator, pulled out food, and started eating anything he could find. When he worried about money, he sat at the table and ate as he talked about finances. All through your years of growing up, you saw that type of behavior. Although you were not consciously learning a lesson in life, your father was teaching you. His actions were saying, "See, when you have problems, eat something. You'll feel better." He was ringing the bell for you, but you were not aware of the effects of his behavior.

By the time you were in high school, you didn't notice that you stuffed yourself with food while you studied for a final exam. No one pointed out that when you faced tension, stress, problems, or difficulties, you automatically reached for something to chew on. You didn't even think about your "need to eat." When you went on a date and you didn't eat heavily before, during, and afterward, you felt uncomfortable.

Even now as an adult, when you have to meet someone in an unfamiliar situation, you fortify yourself with a doughnut and coffee, and you tell yourself, "I'm relaxing a little first." And you do feel a little better! Two helpings of chocolate ice cream enable you to get through the process of balancing the checkbook.

Obviously, the outside influences that are triggers for you may not be for others. Aside from normal hunger, anytime you feel a craving for food, you can know that some outside influence has triggered an automatic response. Your craving is evidence of something going on inside your brain. It's not that you need the food for survival, but your brain says, "You can't cope unless you eat."

At this stage, you probably don't know your triggers. But you can learn that "something" happens before your brain chemicals cry out for more food.

1. Responses to triggers occur automatically. You do not control them by exerting willpower. (You tried that in the past, and it didn't work.)

2. No matter how much you say you don't want to overeat, at this point, you have little choice. Once the trigger is pulled, the automatic response takes over and controls you.

3. This automatic eating may be in response to a trigger that developed when you were a child.

4. The good news is that because it was learned, the automatic response can be unlearned.

5. If you understand this, you can free yourself from guilt feelings because of your dependence on food. You can learn healthy ways to disengage your trigger mechanism.

♥ ♥ ♥

I want you to figure out your triggers. Exercise 1 deals with emotional triggers—emotions that trigger automatic responses in your brain. Read each question carefully. If the emotion is something you frequently or regularly feel, check the yes box.

As you read, if you get a sense of "Aha! That's me!" mark it yes. If you recognize yourself, you are getting to your triggers. You are admitting to yourself, "Whenever I feel a particular way, I eat." Only by being honest with yourself can you make the changes to eliminate your triggering emotions.

———————————————— ♥ ♥ ♥ ————————————————

Vital facts about myself: I acknowledge that I have specific emotional triggers that cause me to overeat. I commit myself to discover these triggers and eliminate them.

———————————————— ♥ ♥ ♥ ————————————————

Read the questions in Exercise 1, and answer yes or no.

EXERCISE 1:
DISCOVERING TRIGGER EMOTIONS

1. Do you eat when you feel bored? Nothing is going on. None of your friends are around. You just can't think of anything you want to put your energy into right now. At this time, does your mind turn to food?   Yes □   No □

2. Do you eat when you are depressed? Do you eat when things are not going right, when you have a sense of uselessness, or when you feel disappointed or let down?   Yes □   No □

3. Do you eat when you feel a low-energy level? At work, as you think about your day ahead, do you inwardly groan? Do you wish you could just do nothing? Do you feel you just can't get enough energy unless you have something to crank you up?   Yes □   No □

4. Do you eat when you feel rejected? You often feel people don't care or don't respond to you. They ignore you or don't give credit for what you do. Whenever you get romantically interested, the person turns you down flat.   Yes □   No □

5. Do you eat when you feel lonely? Do you often feel empty? You may not be able to identify your empty feeling, but you don't feel quite right. You feel there is no one

out there really for you and you're emotionally all
alone.   Yes ☐   No ☐

6. Do you eat when you experience mood changes?
Sometimes it could be during the premenstrual or
menstrual cycle. We now know that men go through
emotional cycles, too. Do you feel extremely happy and
then, for seemingly no reason, you're in a blue mood? Are you
up and down emotionally?   Yes ☐   No ☐

7. Do you eat when you feel anxious? It is an undefined
gnawing inside. You're concerned, maybe worried, but
unable to figure out exactly what bugs you. You have a sense
of foreboding that something isn't right, and you're not
sure what that something is.   Yes ☐   No ☐

8. Do you eat when you feel stressed? You feel pressure
because of your finances, your marriage or romantic
situation, the kids, your parents, or your job. You have this
sense of being pushed down, down, down and don't quite
know how to get the load off your back.   Yes ☐   No ☐

9. Do you eat when you feel embarrassed? Are you
insecure? Are you shy and easily made uncomfortable
with the way people look at you or talk to you? You don't
volunteer for anything because you're sure you'll
embarrass yourself or others.   Yes ☐   No ☐

10. Do you eat when you feel afraid? Are you afraid of
failing? Of not having enough money? Of losing your job?
Of your parents and their involvement in your life? Or your
fear may not be that clearly defined, but you don't try
anything new. Are you too uncomfortable to go to a new
restaurant or try a new kind of food at a place you
regularly eat? Are you afraid to fly in planes? Shop in a
crowded store?   Yes ☐   No ☐

11. Do you eat when you feel inadequate? Do you feel
you have to behave like somebody you're not? Do you
feel inadequate just being who you are? Are you afraid
that others will know you're incompetent even though
you may have a top job? Do you have this nagging sense
that no matter what you do, it's never quite good
enough?   Yes ☐   No ☐

12. Do you eat when you feel excited or happy? Do you keep on feeling that life is party time? Does your world revolve around Friday when you've got money so you can celebrate?   Yes ☐   No ☐

13. Do you eat when you feel angry or irritated? No matter what goes on, do you feel a quiet hostility toward others or toward your work? People have called you a grouch or a sourpuss. Are you just angry at life, feeling things haven't gone right for you? Do people keep doing little things to upset you?   Yes ☐   No ☐

14. Do you eat after you have experienced nightmares? Do you wake up with nightmares? Do you hate to sleep because you awaken scared and shaky?   Yes ☐   No ☐

15. Do you eat when you feel physical pain? Are you in constant or recurring pain? Do you have an ongoing condition such as low back pain, headaches, glaucoma, or sinusitis? Do you constantly look for something to alleviate the pain?   Yes ☐   No ☐

16. Do you eat when you feel an excessive amount of energy? Sometimes is your energy level just too high? Sometimes are you unable to unwind?   Yes ☐   No ☐

17. Do you eat when you feel guilty? Do you struggle with feelings of guilt over what you've done or didn't do in the past? For example, you let down your parents, God, your spouse and kids, or your friends. You work hard, but you feel guilty because you don't work harder. Do you feel guilty because there are problems in the home and you can't say the right words or intervene to make everything okay?   Yes ☐   No ☐

18. Do you eat when you feel proud of yourself or when you feel superior? You want to be somebody important and special. When you compare yourself with others, you feel smug or superior. At the end of the workday, you're still charged up while your coworkers are worn out so you feel you're a better worker. You own a Porsche, and your best friend has "only" a Chevrolet.   Yes ☐   No ☐

19. Do you eat when you feel helpless? Regardless of what

you do, you feel that it won't make any difference. You say, "My situation isn't going to get any better."   Yes☐   No☐

20. Do you eat when you feel confused? Where do you turn? Should you change jobs? Get a divorce? Move to Hawaii? No matter which way you turn, you get no answers or those you get turn out to be wrong. You say often, "I just don't know what to do."   Yes ☐   No ☐

21. Do you have triggers of which you are aware but were not mentioned?   Yes ☐   No ☐

If so, list those triggers:

_____

_____

_____

Scoring:
The *number* of triggers isn't important. What is important is that you recognize your triggers. Go back and find each item with a check mark in the yes box. Those emotions are probably triggers for you.

When you have finished the exercise, talk to your support person. Share your responses. Look at your emotional state when you turn to food. Let your support person help you zero in on your primary emotional triggers. List those triggers.

_____

_____

_____

_____

_____

16

♥

Situational Triggers

"No social activities for me for at least the next two months," Myra told her friends. For Myra, social activities referred primarily to bowling and square dancing.

When one of her friends pressed her, Myra said, "I can control my eating except in those two places. It's only then that I blow my diet and gain back everything I've worked for two weeks to get rid of."

At the time Myra didn't know about triggers, especially situational triggers, but she had figured out something important: Certain activities or environments triggered her need to eat.

In the last chapter, I had you look at emotions that trigger your overeating. Now I want you to look at the context—the situations—where your bell gets rung and you automatically turn to food.

Situations that might be triggers include parties, outings, dates, or any activity where you interact with others. You go to a church function. You're horrified that you fill your plate four times. Your boss or supervisor wants you to attend an important party. Afterward you realize that you're the only person who took seconds on the food. Other potential situational triggers occur when you are not around others. In fact, when someone else is around, overeating may not be a problem for you. But when you're alone in a particular situation (at supper time, for example), you can't stop until you feel stuffed.

I've just described several situations. Any of them could

cause you to feel a particular emotion that might then lead you to turn to food. Generally, the emotion is the actual trigger. But when the emotion is frequently linked to a particular situation for you, it's more helpful to think of the situation as the trigger.

Read the questions in Exercise 2, and answer yes or no.

EXERCISE 2:
DISCOVERING TRIGGER SITUATIONS

1. Do you want to eat when you think about death? Whenever a loved one is ill or you are ill, do you begin to think about death, and it scares you so much that you want to cover up the pain? You eat. You want to get rid of that negativity, and food does that for you.   Yes ☐   No ☐

2. Do you want to eat when you think about money? It isn't a fear of having too much (although that happens to some people), but this feeling of hunger comes over you whenever you're in a situation involving finances. You worry that you

- won't have enough to pay your bills.
- won't be able to provide for your family.
- won't be successful because you associate money with success.
- won't be able to depend on your company's pension policy, the government's Social Security system, or any retirement plan.

Yes ☐   No ☐

3. Do you want to eat when you think about losing your job? You have a daily fear that your company will close or that you'll be fired. You frequently worry about whether you'll have a job in a few months or in three years. You worry about whether you can keep up with the demands of your position. You hear about company cutbacks and hostile takeovers, and you are fearful about your company's survival.   Yes ☐   No ☐

4. Do you want to eat when you think about promotion? Are you afraid that if you turn this one down, you will

never have another chance for advancement? Are you afraid that you've been promoted to the point that you're beyond your ability and you'll be found out?   Yes ☐   No ☐

5. Do you want to eat when you think about intimacy or your sexual performance? Do you feel that you're not romantic enough? That you don't have your sexual needs met? Perhaps you feel as if your spouse is asking you to perform so that sex is a super experience every time, and you're worried that you just can't meet those expectations. Do you associate your first sexual experience with food? When you don't have food before or after a sexual experience, do you feel you'll be an inadequate partner?   Yes ☐   No ☐

6. Do you want to eat when you think about failure? Have you hesitated to volunteer or get involved in activities because you may fail? If your relationships aren't perfect and happy, do you feel as if you have failed? If there are serious conflicts among siblings or family members, do you think you have personally failed for not solving the problems?   Yes ☐   No ☐

7. Do you want to eat when you think about your past? Does it hold feelings of shame? Do you still feel bad about your childhood and family situation? Particularly, do you think of something you did wrong that still haunts you? If your parents are dead, was there something you needed to tell them, but you were not able to do so? Is there something you did in your past that no one ever knew about, yet you're frequently afraid that others will find out, that it will belittle you in their eyes and expose you for being a lesser person?   Yes ☐   No ☐

8. Do you want to eat when you think about being physically hurt or harmed? Are you afraid to be alone in your home? Do you think of strangers as possible rapists, murderers, or thieves?   Yes ☐   No ☐

9. Do you want to eat when you think about your physical appearance? Are you afraid to look attractive? Are you fearful of being too attractive? Or because you're not attractive, perhaps you think people won't see you for who you are?   Yes ☐   No ☐

10. Do you want to eat when you think about your identity? Are you afraid to find out who you really are? Are you afraid that deep inside you think of yourself as a bad person? A negative or dishonest individual? Do you worry that if people find out who you really are inside, they will despise you?   Yes ☐   No ☐

11. Do you want to eat when you think about your sexual identity? Are you afraid others will think you're gay? Are you afraid of who you are? Do you feel confused about your sexual identity?   Yes ☐   No ☐

12. Do you want to eat when you think about participating in certain activities? I know of several people who judge themselves as hosts based on how much food is available at their confirmations, weddings, and similar events. They are aware that many people automatically overeat at these "celebration" activities, and as hosts they want to make sure there is enough food for everyone.   Yes ☐   No ☐

13. Do you want to eat when you think about stress at work? Even if you enjoy your job, are you concerned about the stress level? Do you feel the position holds too much tension, and you're sometimes afraid that you may crack under the strain? Every time you turn around, do you feel new problems have been laid on your shoulders?   Yes ☐   No ☐

14. Do you want to eat when you need to sleep? Do you not sleep enough? Will your mind not shut off when you try to sleep? Are you afraid of nightmares or of falling asleep?   Yes ☐   No ☐

15. Is your desire to eat related to your menstrual or emotional cycle? Do your moods change drastically? Do you crave food and believe it will help you feel better?   Yes ☐   No ☐

16. Can you think of other situations that trigger your eating?   Yes ☐   No ☐

If so, list those situations:

_____

_____

Scoring:

Again, the number of triggers isn't important. What is important is that you recognize your triggers. Go back and find each item with a mark in the yes box. Those situations are probably triggers for you.

After you have completed this exercise, I'd like you to

- discuss the results with your support person.
- select your most difficult situations.
- list those situations. (Use as few or as many spaces as you need.)

_____

_____

_____

_____

_____

- look at the specific things that will help you personally change some situations so they no longer trigger your desire for food. You're going to change your situations from creating emotional triggers. Emotions are the triggers that make you reach for food in just the same way the bell made the dogs salivate in Pavlov's experiment.

♥ ♥ ♥

Vital facts about myself: I have specific trigger situations that cause me to overeat. I commit myself to discover these triggers and eliminate them.

♥ ♥ ♥

17

♥

Preventing the Trigger Response

♥ ♥ ♥

Vital facts about myself: I am aware of the emotions and situations that trigger my misuse of food. Because I am aware, I can change.

♥ ♥ ♥

In the previous chapter, you selected situations that created emotions that got you in trouble. Now you can consider methods to prevent trigger responses. After you read about the six methods, check yes in Exercise 3 on the steps you need to take to prevent trigger responses.

1. PREPARE FOR SOCIAL EVENTS

Social events—anything from going out with others or being involved in events to interacting with your spouse—can pull your trigger. So, let's say you've been invited to a social gathering with a group of people. It is held somewhere you've not been before. You have already decided that you don't want to eat or drink there. What else can you do? You have several options.

First, as soon as you get there, say to the host, "I'm on a special eating plan, so I hope you'll understand if I appear to be a picky eater." Not many people can be so candid. If you can,

I urge you to say it up front. Once you've made your position clear, your discomfort will decrease.

A second option is to say to the host as soon as you get there, "I may have to leave early. I appreciate the invitation, but..." Offer a true, reasonable excuse. The rest of the statement can be as simple as: "A number of other things are going on. I didn't want to miss this event, though." You don't need to say more than that.

If you prepare an excuse and inform your host at the beginning of the evening,

- you can leave whenever you choose.
- you will feel more comfortable.
- you have done something positive for yourself.
- you are not relying on food.

By the way, when you reach a level of discomfort, you can ask to use the phone and say, "I need to make a quick phone call to see if I can stay." Arrange with someone to be available for you to call. Just doing this action will give you the space to decide whether you want to stay. If you feel you can, come back and say, "I can stay."

On the other hand, if your thoughts are filled with food or you're becoming anxious or nervous, you can say, "Thanks so much for inviting me, but I must leave now."

A third option is to enlist your spouse or a friend to be supportive. Tell this person your guidelines, what you want him or her to do, and how he or she can help you in the situation. That person will need to stay close to you during the social event.

A fourth option is to avoid the event altogether. If it's early in your food-recovery program, you may choose to say that you have other plans and cannot attend. You don't have to explain your other plans to avoid an intensely uncomfortable situation.

2. PLAN YOUR FINANCES

Perhaps you struggle with your finances. You may need to talk to somebody. A support person who handles money well would be ideal. Or you may turn to your spouse, a parent, a friend, or your pastor. Select someone you trust who will help you move out of your stressful situation and will help you set up a budget.

When you work on budgeting your money, figure out your obligations and expenses, and divide up the money. If you come up short so that your income won't stretch to include all your needs and expenses, you can decide how to cut back on what you spend, or you can decide how to earn more money.

If your option is to increase your income, and you are sure you won't turn into a compulsive workaholic, you may want to do that. However, it is usually easier and less stressful to make cuts in the way you spend your money.

If you still have problems and can't resolve your financial matters alone or with the person to whom you have turned, you may consider asking a third party. Or you may choose to consult with people who specialize in helping individuals budget their funds.

3. DISCUSS YOUR NEEDS

"I need..."

"I want..."

Many food-dependent people have difficulty making these declarations. One reason for their misuse of food is their inability or unwillingness to express a need.

You can help yourself immensely if you practice starting sentences with those words. Of course, you may not get what you want or need, but at least you are stating it clearly. This simple step can be a breakthrough for you.

If you have problems in your job, focus on one small thing you need that your boss or supervisor can reasonably give and is likely to give. Take an easy problem first so that you can learn to do it. Go to that person and say, "I need...," and set forth what you need in one simple, direct statement. Here are some examples:

- "I need a week's notice before you want a big report." (Previously you had only a single day's notice.)
- "I need for you to explain once again the way you want me to..."

- "I need compliments when I do something right or before you correct me."

To your spouse or a close friend, you may choose to say,

- "I need your support and encouragement."
- "I need your praise when I do something right or thoughtful."
- "I need to feel loved. I want you to hold me."

If you practice on your friends and express your needs, you learn to feel comfortable and able to do it elsewhere.

4. MAKE AN APPOINTMENT WITH YOUR PHYSICIAN

You may have some physically induced issues. Maybe you need to make a physician's appointment. If you are experiencing some form of sexual dysfunction, it may be a wise idea to check with your physician. However, be aware that despite your improved eating plan, you may encounter this dysfunction for a period of time. If you are within the first couple of months of your recovery, you may want to give it more time. If it has been more than two months, you may want to get a medical checkup to find out if there is a physiological cause.

If you're in constant pain, you may want to go to a physician to find out what is creating the pain and the issue associated with the pain.

Sleep disturbances can be an underlying factor of psychological or medical illnesses, or can be caused by them. Again, consider setting up a medical appointment. Food can alter your sleeping patterns, especially in the early weeks of your recovery; you may want to give it more time.

If you have PMS—premenstrual syndrome—with the accompanying symptoms of mood swings and irritability and you feel your emotions are out of control, get medical help first.

5. TALK TO A MINISTER OR COUNSELOR

If you're having trouble over pornography, spiritual difficulties, or involvement with cults, you would do well to talk to either a counselor or a pastor. Tell the person exactly what is going on. Enlist aid in helping you make changes.

6. CHANGE YOUR PRIORITIES

In changing your priorities, here are some things to consider.

First, you may want to change your priorities concerning relationships. This may lead you to change friends because

- they are involved with the situations where you struggle most with food.
- they may not be sympathetic and supportive of your changes. (After all, they were your friends *before* you made changes.)
- they may not be true friends. You associated with them, leaned on them, or allowed them to lean on you, but the relationship was not healthy.

Second, you may decide to change your priorities concerning your job. Perhaps the job causes you problems and places you under constant stress. You may decide that having fewer problems and less stress is more important than staying in the position.

Third, maybe you have to deal with some health issues. You have to make a decision to take care of yourself and not do some activities you've done in the past. You're not going to live the life-style you've been pursuing. You're going to change your priorities on health.

If you can think of any other steps that might be helpful, please add them as number seven on Exercise 3.

On each item in Exercise 3, indicate whether or not this is a step you need to take by checking yes or no.

EXERCISE 3:
PREVENTING THE TRIGGER RESPONSE

1. Prepare for social events.   Yes ☐   No ☐

2. Plan my finances.   Yes ☐   No ☐

3. Discuss my needs.   Yes ☐   No ☐

4. Make an appointment
   with my physician.   Yes ☐   No ☐

5. Talk to a minister or
   counselor.   Yes ☐   No ☐

6. Change my priorities.   Yes ☐   No ☐

7. _____

Now that you've examined the six methods to prevent trigger responses, meet with your support person. Discuss Exercise 3, and get a reality check. Ask, "Can you add anything more? Help me develop these ideas. Show me how to strengthen myself and build a healthy offensive plan not to let these trigger situations hit."

Eventually you're going to program your brain so that when the bell goes off, you will get a different response. But for now, select the most important steps that you can take to prevent the trigger response.

18

— ♥ —

Thought Towers

Sara was raised in a family where she never felt as if she did anything right. She learned as a child that when she felt inadequate, eating eased those painful feelings. Later as an adult, she developed a thought tower that worked like this:

1. Sara had a minor disagreement with her husband.
2. Sara thought about the situation. She then felt inadequate. After all, if she was the kind of wife she should be, there would never be any arguments. She must have done something wrong.
3. Sara's feelings of inadequacy caused her serotonin levels to drop.
4. The drop in serotonin brought about a biological response—depression.
5. The low serotonin and depression brought about an automatic response—she ate.
6. Eating increased Sara's serotonin, decreased her depression, and provided her with a reward—she felt better.
7. Because of her reward, the cycle would start all over again whenever anything went wrong.

Sara's problem began with her thoughts. Once she started on a new cycle, everything went into automatic action. She was able to make changes only after she could identify her thoughts and see their effects.

That's the point of this illustration. I want you to learn to identify your thoughts. It is not only *what* you think but *how* you think that has gotten you to misuse food in the past.

Here's a quick review about neurochemistry and thoughts to show you why you should identify your thoughts.

1. You start with a conflict. (That conflict can be a thought or a situation.)
2. The conflict creates or enhances the thoughts.
3. The thoughts bring about a neurochemical change.
4. Your chemical changes in the brain bring about or cause an emotion (i.e., stress, anxiety, fear).
5. The emotion causes you to react. You behave in a particular way. You overeat. (In the illustration, Sara reached for food.)
6. The action you take creates or provides a reward, even though it may be a negative reward.
7. After you act, the chemicals go back to what your brain considers its normal level—your baseline transmission. You may have done this so often, your baseline transmission level may actually be abnormal. (In the illustration, Sara felt better after she ate and her neurochemicals balanced again.)
8. You no longer feel the emotion of stress, anxiety, or fear. Or if you do, it's at a less intense level.

DEFINING TERMS

Previously, I've talked about Pavlov's experiment, particularly about the dogs, the food, the bell, and the salivation. Once a bell went off, the dogs' action (or response) became automatic. In the eight progressive steps above, the bell went off with the conflicting thoughts (Step 2—it is often difficult, and unnecessary, to determine whether the thought causes the internal conflict or vice versa). That's all it takes. If you can envision your thoughts as the bell, you can see how this example applies to you and your misuse of food. The ringing bell (conflicting thoughts) makes the chemicals *automatically* respond, which, in turn, causes an *automatic* behavior to kick in.

Already you can see that if you are to make permanent changes in your eating habits, you have to prevent the bell from ringing. That's what we want to work on now. You're going to look at thought triggers—specific thoughts that I refer to as *thought towers*.

Another illustration may help you understand what I mean by thought towers. You have a set of building blocks that interlock. You stack them up and make a tower. If you have ever done this, you know that as you continue to add blocks, the tower gets top-heavy. If you continue, at some point adding *one* block will make the entire tower collapse.

However, the *last* block doesn't bring down the tower. It isn't the fault of any single block. The accumulated weight of all the blocks causes the tower to fall.

Think of your thoughts as building blocks in erecting a tower. The thoughts that arise when you encounter a conflict generally consist of a theme. In Sara's case, her problems went back to a theme of inadequacy.

A second term I want to define is a *compulsive theme*. You have a psychological need—a need so important that you must satisfy it. It's not a choice. It's a need that you cannot ignore or deny. In your case, you satisfy that need through compulsive overeating.

As I have previously pointed out, themes vary. If your theme is power, you overeat to calm or satisfy that need. When you overeat, you don't solve the issue. If you solved the issue, you would no longer have a compulsive form of behavior (your overeating). If power is your theme, eating smooths over your burning compulsion to exert power. If you *need* to control the behavior of everyone in your house—and control is one form of power—what do you do? At this stage of your recovery, you have two obvious choices:

1. You take total control of the thoughts and actions of your family members. Doing this is impossible, of course.
2. You overeat, which dulls your need. Food temporarily lessens your power need.

Let's try another example involving a thought tower.

1. You're under heavy stress on the job.
2. You feel a lot of stress at home because your spouse won't help with the household chores.
3. Your parents phone you regularly. You feel they demand more of your time and attention. The pressure on you increases.
4. You feel your children aren't responding to you. You're particularly worried because they don't seem to have any real faith in God, no matter what you say or do.

Those are four separate issues. *Or are they separate?* Read the list again. What if they are connected by a single theme? Maybe the theme is one of feeling inadequate.

If you have trouble feeling comfortable with who you are or feeling adequate, it shows up in all four problems. You're uncomfortable with relationships because you don't think anybody really loves you. You have such a low sense of self-esteem, you don't feel lovable.

Suppose your theme of adequacy, particularly in your relationships, is the common theme that goes in building your tower. That means you can deal with your job all you want; you may find some helpful ways to get along better with your coworkers. In the meantime, you have three other blocks—all of them demanding attention *right now.* Or if you deal with your children or tackle the issue of your parents, you have the same results.

You make the same mistake that most people do when it comes to addictive and compulsive behavior. You attack a symptom and don't get to the root. Instead of struggling with the four actual situations that overwhelm you, suppose you tried another perspective. If you got back to the core of your problem, you could work on that solution. It would then carry over into all parts of your life.

Let's say you decide on the core issue: I feel that I am not lovable or adequate. You make a concerted effort to change that attitude about yourself. You tackle one problem. When you solve that problem, you realize that it affects your relationships at work, with your spouse, your children, and your parents.

I want you to examine a specific thought tower. If you deal with one compulsive theme—one overpowering need—you won't have to keep on trying to fix every little problem that erupts in your life. You won't have to feel like a failure because you can't change everything and console yourself with more food.

It becomes increasingly difficult and nonproductive to deal with problem after problem after problem when you've never dealt with the real issue. Or medically, I could say it's like treating the symptom without ever discovering the disease. For example, if your eyes are sore, you buy eye drops. Every time your eyes feel strained or sore, you use the drops. You will never be cured because the problem isn't the soreness. Your problem is that you need eyeglasses so you won't strain your eyes. The *result* of the problem of poor eyesight is strain, hence the soreness. If your doctor prescribes glasses, you no longer need the eye drops. You have moved from the symptom to the care of the problem.

Let's look further into thoughts. Ask yourself, Are my thoughts facts? Or are my thoughts only my perceptions?

For example, Frank has a thought that says he is stupid. Is he stupid? Or is it more correct to say that Frank *feels* stupid? That does not say if he is bright or dull. If Frank goes through life thinking he is stupid (and let's say he is extremely intelligent), he is bound to have problems because he believes something about himself that is not true.

Here is a principle: The majority of thoughts that get you in trouble are not facts; they are only your perceptions. Your perceptions may be inaccurate.

Think about this imaginary conversation:

You say, "My husband doesn't love me."

"How do you know that?" I ask.

"I don't feel loved."

"You don't feel loved," I answer, "but that doesn't mean you are not loved, does it? You are taking a feeling and calling it a fact."

Thoughts and feelings involve the way in which you were taught about yourself. You accepted them as true, but they might or might not have been true. Are any of these statements "facts" you accepted about yourself?

- I am lazy.
- I am worthless.
- I can't do anything right.
- I will never amount to anything.
- I am so dumb with math, I can't even balance a checkbook.
- I am not pretty like my sister (or handsome like my brother).

Any of the statements may sound like a "fact." In reality, they are only your thoughts—how you perceive yourself.

Here's an example. You had a beautiful sister. When you were young, she got all the recognition for her pretty features. "Your sister is so pretty," people told you. You interpreted those words to mean that you were not pretty because you didn't get those compliments. You might have been quite beautiful, and it was so obvious that no one said much. Or perhaps people told your sister about how pretty you were.

Through the years, you stored up in your mind that you weren't good-looking. No one ever said you were plain or ugly, but you assumed it because you didn't get compliments. Or perhaps someone said it once in anger, and you accepted the statement as fact. You stored those untrue, angry words as truth.

Every time you are called upon in your brain to pick up stored memory, you pick up things such as:

- I'm not good enough.
- I'm not pretty enough.
- I'm ugly.
- Everybody knows I'm ugly, and people laugh at me.

You have such thoughts now because you stored those thoughts chemically in your brain.

What if you were told that you weren't a nice person, that you didn't do things right, and that you weren't smart? (Frequently, that message is sent when parents don't give enough praise to their children.) Those messages were stored in your brain. You took on an art project for school, and you worked hard on it. When you showed it to your parents, your father said, "It doesn't look much like a cow to me," and your mother lectured you on perspective. After that, no matter what you did, you knew it wasn't good enough.

Now you're an adult, and you have developed a low sense of self-esteem. You are thirty-five years old, and you have been asked to give a speech to a group of important people. Doing a good job requires a high level of self-esteem. You begin to develop the project. As you work, intellectually you know that you're doing your best and you are good in your field. Otherwise, you wouldn't have been asked to give the speech.

When the day arrives for you to speak, doubts fill your mind. You wonder if you're going to do it well enough. You wonder if the audience will like you. Your mind is filled with thoughts of making mistakes, forgetting what to say, dropping your notes, or tripping on electric cords. You get slightly sick to your stomach, and you fear that you're running a fever.

Why all these negative reactions? Because of what has happened in your past. You are called upon to exert positive self-esteem. You can't do that because you have stored up the "facts" that you're not good enough. You feel inferior, and your thoughts cluster around all the things you can or may do wrong. Now you can understand why you have to identify those thoughts. Even though you believe them, they may not be based on reality. You may be more than good enough, even excellent. But you will never know unless you do something to find out.

FIGURING OUT THOUGHT PROCESSES

Exercise 4 (on page 171) asks you to identify your two most significant needs related to your thought towers. As you read the six discussed here, consider how you will answer. (You may think of others not included here.)

1. Your need to feel adequate

How often do you develop thoughts that sound like these?

- "I don't know if I'm going to be good enough."
- "Why did I ever think I could do this?"
- "I'm really going to blow it this time."

Your need to feel adequate is essential for your recovery. In Exercises 2 and 3, you saw how your emotions feed into fear of social situations and affect virtually every aspect of your life. If you think about those situations, they have to do with feelings of inadequacy.

Find out if that's your theme. It will be easier to fight one thought, a feeling of inadequacy, than a variety of situations.

2. Your need for approval and acceptance

You may do your job remarkably well, but if no one tells you, how do you know how good it is?

A graduate student named Jeff was extremely bright. He came from a family of highly intelligent people. He said that until he took the Graduate Record Examination, he had assumed that "I was adequate. Not really dumb and not particularly smart."

Everybody needs affirmation for doing a good job. Some people have advocated self-talk. You stand in front of the mirror, stare at your reflection, and say, "I am attractive." There is nothing wrong with that, but it doesn't go far enough. You need people to affirm you in some way. When you work hard, you need someone to recognize your efforts. Or when you do something well, just doing it well isn't good enough; you need the praise.

If you're constantly caught up in situations where you receive no approval and no praise, you'll continue to yearn for them. You'll feel rejected because you didn't get the positive affirmations you need.

3. Your need for love

All of us need to be loved. But is your need to the point that you change who you are and try to do things to get people to love you? Do you feel no love from yourself, from God, or from other people? You just don't feel like a lovable person.

A psychologist named Abraham Maslow constructed what he called a hierarchy of needs. He said that when people are hungry or thirsty, they have no other needs. But once they get food or water, the next need is the need for protection or safety. Once they feel their basic needs are provided for, they need to be loved and to feel that they belong. When they know they are loved, they're ready for the next step, which is developing self-esteem.

Many people can't get beyond the need for love and don't develop self-esteem. Even on the lecture circuit, I meet well-known individuals who smile, know how to say the right things to their audience, and give the impression that they feel loved and accepted. But I've been able to watch them when they step off the platform and see their other side. They're aggressive and demanding. They make persons around them unhappy. They're obsessive about certain things. All of this happens, I believe, because they have never truly felt loved.

4. Your need to be understood

Ever feel that nobody understands you? That nobody realizes what you're going through? Nobody understands the way things are, and it's frustrating to you because you look around and say, "I've been doing all these things and nobody cares." Or you do something and think you've done a great job, but nobody gives you recognition. So you're sitting there saying, "Why don't they understand what I've done?"

5. Your need to be appreciated

Or you could say this is the need to be appreciated for what you do. If you're like most people, you want to feel that you make a difference somewhere in the world. You want to feel that someone needs you, and you can provide something financially, emotionally, or spiritually.

6. Your need to be needed

You need to be needed, to have someone else depend on you. When you're needed, you have a reason to work through hassles. You're helping someone or a cause. You are useful in this life.

♥ ♥ ♥

Vital facts about myself: I am loved. I
am adequate.

♥ ♥ ♥

EXERCISE 4:
IDENTIFYING MY THOUGHT TOWERS

Put an X by your two most significant needs related to your thought towers. You may add others not mentioned.

_____ 1. I need to feel adequate.

_____ 2. I need approval and acceptance.

_____ 3. I need to feel loved.

_____ 4. I need to feel understood.

_____ 5. I need to feel appreciated.

_____ 6. I need to feel needed.

_____ 7. I need _____.

EXERCISE 5:
BUILDING MY TOWERS

As you get stronger and have been free from your food dependency, you're going to be able to identify your thought tower fairly easy. For now you're going to fight the thought by changing the situation—you're preventing the bell from ringing. In time, you will feel adequate, and you will feel approval, love, or whatever you need. You will change the thoughts that create the negative feelings.

1. From Exercises 1 and 2 select the three most important emotions and the three corresponding situations. You're going to build towers.

2. Identify the thoughts that lead to these emotions. Try to be aware of what is happening when the emotions come to you. When you're stressed at work, is it because you need to feel adequate? Maybe the emotion is stress or confusion. Using this illustration, you would fill in Tower 1 this way:

  a) THOUGHT: I need to feel adequate
  b) SITUATION: stress at work
  c) EMOTION: confusion and stress

3. Do the exercise, completing one tower for each of the three emotions.

Tower 1

a) THOUGHT:
b) SITUATION:
c) EMOTION:

Tower 2

a) THOUGHT:
b) SITUATION:
c) EMOTION:

Tower 3

a) THOUGHT:
b) SITUATION:
c) EMOTION:

4. After you have finished the exercise, share the results with your support person.

19

♥

Changing Your Thoughts

You can change your thoughts. That will keep your tower from falling. Changing your thoughts begins with a two-step process: (1) You recognize where your wrong thinking comes from, and (2) you review the way you have previously looked at your conflicts and yourself. For the rest of this chapter, you're going to focus on identifying your wrong thinking. (In the next chapter you're going to look at the way you see your life—your spiritual outlook.)

Essentially, you have in your thought tower a thought that creates a conflict that creates an emotion that pushes you to do a form of behavior. If you could back up and change your initial thinking, the situation would not create the same negative emotion that it did before.

Let's say that my thought was a feeling of inadequacy, the setting was at work, and the emotion was stress. If I felt adequate, work would no longer create stress, and I could look at my life differently. My work could be a challenge rather than a threat. So my wrong thinking was that I felt inadequate.

To make the changes, I state the new thought: "I feel adequate." I decide that my spouse will provide the support I need. If I have a support person, I include him as well—or another individual who validates me as I work on adequacy. My new response is the ability to relax and walk away from work when I leave at the end of the day.

In Exercise 5, you may have written, "I need to be sexually rewarded." Is that really a need? Or is it more appropriate to

173

write, "I need to be loved"? Or is it perhaps a need to be appreciated or to feel adequate? That's what you have to identify.

EXERCISE 6:
DETERMINING NEW THINKING

Let's work the exercise step by step.

1. Mark off four columns on a sheet of paper. Label them "Wrong Thinking," "New Thought Needed," "Support Needed," and "New Response." In the column "Wrong Thinking," write the things that are wrong. Be as honest with yourself as possible. You may put the following:

- I am inadequate.
- I am not appreciated.
- I am not needed.

2. The new thoughts are going to be positive:

- I am adequate.
- I am appreciated.
- I am needed.

3. Now you need to find support for your new thoughts. There are two ways to look at this. One way is called feedback, and the other is backtrack.

In feedback you describe your situation, such as your sexuality issue or your work issue, to your support person. You say, "You know, I think this relates to my feelings of inadequacy (or whatever fits)." You discuss it. Your support person gives you a response—an opinion—which is feedback.

You backtrack when you look for similar or related situations in your life. You may finally say, "I remember when I was really stressed at work before. The boss didn't respond to me right away, and I felt that I wasn't important and that my work was inadequate. When she did speak, she was curt with me. So I began to get fearful of holding on to my position. That fits, doesn't it? That's touching on the matter of adequacy."

Ask your support person to help you backtrack. The person

may need to probe and push, but you can backtrack if you're willing to do it. The support may mean, "I can't get approval for what I've done for my boss, but I want to get my approval elsewhere." Perhaps you feel that your boss never approves of anything you do.

I remember the first time I wrote an article that I intended to send to a journal for publication. Before sending it away, I handed it to one of my close friends. "Read this article," I said as I handed it to him.

A few days later he brought the papers back and said, "Joel, that was a good article. Where did you have it published?"

"I haven't published it yet," I said.

"Oh," he said, not sounding very impressed.

Without intending to, my friend was saying that unless I gave a public performance (had my article published), it wasn't worth much.

Another friend wanted to read it, so I gave him a copy. He called me on the phone: "This is phenomenal! Great insight. This is neat, and I love it." There was no performance associated with the article. He was supporting me for working on the article, for getting my thoughts together, and for thinking concisely and clearly. The other friend would not have been a good support person for me.

As you move into backtrack and feedback, you may choose not to use the same support person. Or perhaps you get your best support when you get quiet, and you pray or contemplate. Or a family member may give you what you need.

At this time, ask yourself, Is my support person supportive? Or do I have somebody that I'm not comfortable with? There is no better time than now to make changes as you get into deeper issues. You may also want to ask yourself, Do I need additional support?

4. Now you're ready for the new responses. How do you want to respond?

I want you to write a new response. At first it will be a determination, a goal and not a reality. Each day as you repeat your new response, it will become more real to you.

I'll walk through this with you. Let's go back to the situation with sexual performance and feeling inadequate.

Your wrong thinking is I am inadequate. Your thought tower showed you your need to feel adequate. The emotion is anger. You engaged in sex with your spouse when you didn't really want to, so now you feel used. This is anger.

Your new thought is I am adequate.

You go to your support person, perhaps your spouse. You discuss your need to feel adequate before any sexual activity takes place. The way you feel adequate is for your spouse to treat you with respect. One way to do that is to discuss your sexual needs as well as your spouse's needs.

Your new response is enjoyment without anger. Your thought process is going to feel adequate: "My spouse is going to respect me. I will have a positive feeling."

I hope you can now see why it's important for you to backtrack and go through wrong thinking in the past. You need to be aware of what you absorbed or were taught and whether it was true.

SOMETHING FOR YOU TO
THINK ABOUT

Get into the habit of focusing on your trigger issues. Are you making some changes in the situations so you're not getting the same triggers? Have you identified them? Are you seeing new triggers? Trigger identification is a process. You will see more and more triggers at work in your life. Once you are aware, you can say, "Okay, now I understand these particular triggers. I can change my situations."

You're going to have thought towers—positive and negative. Examine the negative thought towers and change them to the positive. If you change them, you will also effectively change your emotional responses. Make them positive. That's where peace comes from.

I want you to know this about your new responses:

- The new responses are goals.
- The new responses are not going to be natural, so you must work at them.
- It takes time for the new responses to become your first reactions.

20

— ♥ —

Your Spirituality

Spirituality is the subject of this chapter. If you're still in the early phase of recovery, you're probably going to say, "I don't want to deal with any of this religious stuff. I want to get to the important part of my life."

Spritual recovery *is* an important part of your life. You can't dodge it if you want full recovery. Besides that, spiritual recovery is not easy. Even committed Christians have difficulty placing spirituality as a high priority at this stage. Many people feel burned out with the church or with God. Or they don't know what it's all about. If either description fits you, you need to read this chapter. In fact, from my perspective, this chapter is the most vital one in the book. Although you need a lot of information to reach this chapter, if you understand the concepts here, the others will be easier to understand.

From a spiritual standpoint, food dependency affects

- your relationship with God.
- your ability to give love.
- your ability to accept love.
- your ability to accept others as well as yourself.
- your self-discipline.

As you work through issues of spirituality, you'll be able to

- achieve peace.
- live in a growing relationship with God.

• nurture a wholesome relationship with others.
• enhance a healthy love for yourself.

Earlier I wrote about the three parts of human beings. I've already discussed the physical, which includes a plan for activities and an improved eating program. You have set your goals. You have shared with your support person.

In the emotional area, you focused on thoughts and emotions they trigger as well as the situations that create those emotions. You began to come to grips with emotions such as loneliness, fear, and inadequacies.

Now you are ready to move into the spiritual area.

Here is the basic idea behind spiritual health: If you are alive, you will have conflicts. Life *is* conflict—from within and from without. Some conflicts you feel you can handle, and other kinds you can't. Some conflicts you take personally. What you do with conflicts and how you handle them also decide if they become emotional, physical, or spiritual conflicts.

REMEMBER: A conflict causes a thought.

Frequently, kids come to me and say, "My parents don't love me."

"What makes you say that?" I ask.

I get a variety of answers, but they sound like these:

• "They don't hug me."
• "They don't do anything with me."
• "They don't say they love me."

When I speak to the parents, it usually becomes obvious that they love their kids. That's one reason they brought them to see me. But I also see the problem. It is one of three things:

1. The children misperceive the love.
2. The children are loved but not enough.
3. The children or the parents have unrealistic expectations of the other.

The parents may not be demonstrating love because they're not giving the kids enough of their time. The kids haven't learned to look at the way their parents love, so they can't accept that they are loved.

Most of them don't realize that this issue is spiritual. This realm involves our definition of life; it encompasses issues such as acceptance, love, and adequacy.

Unfortunately, too many people get caught up in the religion and religious questions when I talk about spirituality. I bring up the topic, and I get responses about church attendance, baptism, and offerings, or questions about being more active in the church.

"Put aside those ideas right now. Your first step is to look at the spiritual part of your life and develop spiritual health," I say to them.

But here is the principle I want you to grasp—and you may not readily accept it—in a sense, all conflicts are spiritual. If you can resolve spiritual conflicts, you will have fewer negative thoughts, fewer neurochemical changes, fewer emotional changes, and fewer behavioral changes.

You started to read this book because you became aware of a problem. You said, "I think about food constantly, and I overeat. I don't like overeating." You now have read enough that you know your triggers. You know you eat as an automatic reaction to your bell being rung.

Now you are ready for the next question: How do I keep from ringing the bell? Here is the answer: You need to see yourself as you are. When you see yourself as you are, God and other people are also involved. You cannot separate the three. That reality makes this a spiritual issue.

Let's look at a story in the Bible. One day a lawyer asked Jesus to recite the greatest commandment contained in the law of Moses. Jesus answered,

> "'You shall love the LORD your God with all your heart, with all your soul, and with all your mind.' This is the first and great commandment. And the second is like it: 'You shall love your neighbor as yourself.' On these two commandments hang all the Law and the Prophets" (Matt. 22:37–40).

Although they are familiar verses, many people miss something basic. After Jesus quoted the first commandment, He said, "And the second is like it." He meant, "The second is of the same value or substance." He was saying to His listeners that the great commandment of the Bible comes in three parts. You must totally love God, yourself, and others.

The writer named John made this connection clear:

> Brethren, I write no new commandment to you, but an old commandment which you have had from the beginning. The old commandment is the word which you heard from the beginning. Again, a new commandment I write to you, which thing is true in Him and in you.... He who says he is in the light, and hates his brother, is in darkness until now. He who loves his brother abides in the light, and there is no cause for stumbling in him. But he who hates his brother is in darkness and walks in darkness, and does not know where he is going, because the darkness has blinded his eyes (1 John 2:7–11).

Jesus united God, self, and others by stating the principle of the great commandment. The writer John showed how that works out in a practical way. It is impossible to love God without loving others. It is impossible to love yourself without loving God. The relationship is three-way.

How we live with the three-way relationship depends on our outlook on life. That is, for me, the definition of *spiritual*.

Here are my definitions:

spiritual: the purpose of and responses to life as well as the understanding of self, God, and others

spiritual conflicts: disharmony in any of the three areas of unconditional love, acceptance, and self-discipline

spiritual health: a way of seeing what we are when we understand the strengths of who we are; then we know we can change from what we don't want to be

Understanding your spiritual nature determines who you are, how you see life, and what you can do about making changes. Everything else you will be doing in this book is based on this aspect of spirituality.

Here's the next thing for you to grasp: If you can eliminate or minimize your spiritual conflicts, you can minimize self-destructive behavior. After seeing more than eleven thousand people with compulsive behavior issues, I am convinced that people are self-destructive. They have different methods to bring it about, but they keep going back and setting themselves up to fail in their weakest area.

You have at least one weak area in your life. So do I. That is true for everyone. Where you are weak is where you fight the battles.

If you're honest with yourself, you know your area or areas of weakness. Until you overcome that weakness, you'll fail every time. When the trigger goes off, you automatically turn to food. Others turn to drugs or become workaholics or engage in promiscuous sexual activity.

You can overcome this weakness. You can learn to be aware of it, stay out of situations that make you vulnerable, and find ways to cope without reaching for another slice of chocolate cake.

Before we focus on your problem, reflect on the weak areas of others. When you look down on others for failing in some way, you are despising them for giving in to their weak areas. You've forgotten that you also have been failing in your weak area.

Sometimes the weak area is obvious but not always. Consider these situations:

1. Hugh is the office gossip. He knows everything about everybody—especially the bad news.
2. Agnes has had so many sexual affairs, she doesn't even remember the names of all of the men.
3. Mark volunteers for duties and responsibilities at church. But he procrastinates so long that someone else has to jump in at the last minute and force him to get the job done.
4. Catherine arrives at work before everybody else. She stays longer than anyone else and lets it be known that her life is built around her job. Yet, anyone examining her productivity would know that Catherine accomplishes no more than workers who put in normal work hours.

Sometimes we think we have strong areas that are not actually strong. They are our weak areas that we have learned to protect. We then avoid the real issues as if they don't exist.

Now let's look at spiritual conflict. In my years of working with a large number of individuals, I've condensed the areas of spiritual conflict into three broad categories.

1. ACCEPTANCE

This category emphasizes self-acceptance, but it also embraces the acceptance of others. It is the number one spiritual conflict.

First, we want to consider the *acceptance of others.* Most of us believe we're right. Why do we think we're right and argue our point? Even if we don't argue, we're silently convinced we're correct. I don't know any individuals who argue because they think they're wrong.

How do you know you're right? You begin by considering your life experiences—the circumstances of your life. If you tried to do something one way and you didn't succeed, you decided that it didn't work, that it was wrong. So your brain stored up a message, "It doesn't work this way." However, suppose another person tried it that way and it worked. That person's brain stored up the message, "This is the right way." Although something may be right for one person, it is not necessarily right for you.

Let's say I live in Michigan, and I want to go to Florida. The most direct way is to follow Interstate 75 south. So I tell my friend Tyler, "If you want to go to Florida, you take I-75 all the way. You can drive it in twenty-four hours if you go straight through."

Tyler says, "Naw, I don't want to go that way."

"Do what you want," I argue, "but I'm telling you, it's the best way to go."

Why do I argue that my route is the best? Because it's the most direct way, which makes it the fastest. Based on my personality, I make this equation:

$$fastest = best$$

"Here's a better way," Tyler says. "See, I can drive over to New Jersey, follow the coastline through the Carolinas all the way through Georgia, and then on to Florida. It may take me three or four days, but it will be a quiet, scenic trip."

Tyler has a different set of values. His personality is more laid-back, and time is not a top priority for him. His equation reads:

$$\text{scenic} = \text{best}$$

Tyler and I argue. Who is right? We both are in that we're arguing from our values and priorities. We're also both wrong because each of us assumes that his perspective is the only right way. When I insist, "Going I-75 is the best way," I impose my circumstances and values on Tyler. I have formed my personality from my life experiences. However, I don't recognize that I am arguing from a different set of circumstances. Because I am so focused on myself and my need to be accepted as right, I discount anything Tyler says.

Acceptance of others' viewpoints (which is also acceptance of them) is often difficult. Many conflicts in government, neighborhoods, churches, and even families could be eliminated if this were understood.

One couple argued over the time to eat their evening meal. They had been married for six months, and it was still an issue. "Six o'clock is the time to eat your evening meal," the husband insisted.

"Seven is right," she insisted.

He came from a family where they ate breakfast at 6:00 A.M., lunch exactly at noon, and dinner six hours later. He *assumed* that was the proper way.

His wife, by contrast, came from a home where they usually ate at 7:00 P.M. But sometimes other things got in the way, and dinnertime might be 8:00 P.M. or perhaps occasionally 6:45 P.M.

Once both of them were able to admit, "Well, that's the way I was raised," they could move on to listening to each other. They accepted each other's background, although I don't know the time they agreed on.

Acceptance starts by saying, "I'm not right or wrong in my position. From my viewpoint, this is right. I just don't understand where you're coming from."

Acceptance is not based on

- whether others agree with you.
- whether they change.
- whether they see your viewpoint.

Acceptance is just that—"I accept you, and I approve of you as a person." You have to accept others before they make a change or even if they never make a change.

The second aspect of acceptance is *self-acceptance*. Unless you can accept yourself as you are, you won't be able to change. If you don't accept who you are today, you'll get caught up in defending and justifying who you are. You'll find ways to manipulate others—and yourself—to prove who you are. Only if you accept who you are today do you have the opportunity to change.

And how do you change? You begin by accepting yourself as normal. I want to explain what I mean by *normal*.

Let's say you are an employee of the Silver Star Company. Are you a good employee? If you are, how do you figure that out? You have to look at your work and make a decision.

Would this be a realistic way to judge or decide if you are a good employee? You compare yourself to another employee

- who has not missed a day of work in twenty-five years.
- who constantly works overtime.
- who volunteers for activities to make the workplace a better environment.
- who is the first to volunteer to work on holidays.

I hope you immediately declare, "No!"

Is that a model employee? That person is probably the *ultimate* employee in some people's eyes. But he or she is certainly not a normal employee and may not be a model *person*.

Here's what I mean. Ray is that model employee. He works overtime at least four times a week and is always on call. He has never used all his vacation time. Ray is essentially married to his job. The owner of the company may say, "Ray is the best employee I have."

But look more closely. Ray has a terrible time with human relationships. He hasn't devoted enough time and energy to his family. He isn't happy with what he calls "all the complaining I have to listen to." He simply hasn't made his family a high priority. Although a church member, Ray often heads for work instead. He knows he is "not in a very good relationship with God." He wants to trust God, but he is afraid that if he doesn't work harder and harder, he'll lose his job. So he worries about that every day instead of placing God as a priority.

If you compare yourself with Ray, the ultimate employee, you're not being realistic. (And if you knew the other part of his life, is that the way you would want to be?) The worst part is that when you compare yourself with the best, you come out second. Someone is always better.

Let's say 20 percent of the time you're not a good employee and 80 percent of the time you are. What area are you focusing on? The 20 percent that you fail? Or can you focus on the positive 80 percent?

Where do you focus? On perfection or on reality? If you're married, how do you rate yourself as a spouse? Do you look at yourself and say, "I'm a lousy spouse"? But 90 percent of the time you are an excellent spouse, and 10 percent of the time you're not the best.

Focus on who you are, not on what you're not. You may have a food problem, but that's not who you are. You're a person who has excellent potential if you accept who you are today and know you can change.

Accept yourself based on comparing yourself with the normal or *average,* not the *ultimate.* Look at the average worker in your department. If you perform as well as the average, you have done an acceptable job. That gives you a realistic goal. If there are areas where you are exceptionally good, you may increase your standard. But be cautious.

♥ ♥ ♥

Vital facts about myself: I accept myself as I am. Even when I disagree, I accept others as they are.

♥ ♥ ♥

2. UNCONDITIONAL LOVE

Unconditional love means you love somebody else—regardless. You love your child, parents, spouse, and close friends, regardless of whether they're doing what you want them to.

None of us truly loves unconditionally, but we can set it as a goal. God is the only One who truly loves unconditionally.

To get a sense of your level of unconditional love, consider the following questions:

- Do you say, "I'll love you if you do _____ for me"?
- Do you think or actually tell others, "If you don't do that, I won't like you"?
- Do you love people only when they do things your way?
- Do you withhold love or affection when others behave differently from what you want?

Any answer of yes says your love is conditional.

Can you say this?

- "I love you even though I don't like what you're doing."
- "I love you even though you reject my values and turn to your own."

If you can, that's an expression of unconditional love.

What about unconditional love of yourself? Do you love yourself all the time? Can you look at your reflection in a mirror and make these statements?

- "You know, I like you."
- "You are wonderful just the way you are."
- "So you didn't become the employee of the year. I love you anyway."

Unconditional love of yourself is expressed in the following self-affirmation:

------------------ ♥ ♥ ♥ ------------------

A vital fact about myself: No matter what
I do or say, I love myself.

------------------ ♥ ♥ ♥ ------------------

When you can say to another, "No matter what you do or say, I love you," that is unconditional love.

The best example we have is what we know about God. For me, Paul says this beautifully: "But God demonstrates His own love toward us, in that while we were still sinners, Christ died for us" (Rom. 5:8).

3. SELF-DISCIPLINE

Disciplining yourself is not the same as tensing your muscles and using your willpower when the bell rings. Once the bell rings, the response is already beyond your control. You work in advance. You plan to stop the bell from ringing. Or if you go back to my first story about the Shetland ponies, you work at this by learning to take one shovelful at a time instead of trying to control everything. You take a series of small steps—small acts of self-discipline—and eventually you get the barn cleaned up.

If you faithfully follow your specific programs—exercise, activity, behavioral, and eating—and guard your thought processes, you are making strides in the right direction. You are reprogramming yourself so that the bell doesn't ring for you the way it used to.

21

— ♥ —

Your Spiritual Health

Spiritual health? What does that mean?

The way I use the term, you are spiritually healthy if you are progressing in the three major areas of acceptance, unconditional love, and self-discipline.

- You can speak up for yourself in healthy ways and express your needs.
- You can feel your emotions, but they no longer overpower you.
- You can safely experience anger and then find wholesome ways to resolve it.
- You can forgive hurts and rejection received from others.
- You may experience guilt, but you won't be controlled by it.
- You can feel good about yourself with a high level of self-esteem, which is accompanied by inner peace.
- You can understand that you have a purpose in life, and you'll develop a strong sense of who you are.

As you think about these statements, you may wonder how they are possible to achieve. Right now you may feel helpless, unable to believe that they are within your reach. That's why you need to continue reading. I'm going to show you the best way to develop a spiritual outlook. I'll start by giving you principles that lead to spiritual health.

You are already good enough for God

As a person with food-related problems, you may perceive of God as One who demands, judges, and condemns. Because you didn't meet the divine standards, you felt condemned or at least inadequate.

I caution you not to try to prove anything to God or yourself. Although you may have difficulty accepting this fact, God loves you as you are.

Because of your emotional issues and needs, you probably feel spiritually damaged. It is hard for you to believe that God doesn't condemn you for every little mistake you make. A feeling of being judged and condemned may be one of the major obstacles in your spiritual pathway. You will learn to develop a relationship with God based on His acceptance of you.

♥ ♥ ♥

A vital fact about myself:

God loves me as I am.

♥ ♥ ♥

This feeling of inadequacy is so pervasive that you can't ignore it. No matter how true the reality is, you may not be able to accept it. It makes me think of a man who stands in front of a mirror and looks at himself. "I'm a nice person," he says. As he turns to walk away, he adds, "But I'm ugly."

That's the same thing as approaching God and saying, "I believe You love me," and as you walk away, you say, "But You still want to punish me."

As you continue to grow, I hope your faith will increase. Don't allow yourself to add any statements that begin with "but" when you say or think something positive about yourself.

God is all-loving and all-forgiving

In the church we say that God gives us grace. That means God loves us and forgives us, leads us and cares about us, even though none of us is perfect. That's why it's grace—*undeserved* favor.

God is not just a Higher Power or a great Creator but the God revealed in the Bible

God is personally concerned about and interested in you.

You need to see God, others, and yourself realistically

By now I hope you realize that chemical changes in your brain have affected the way you perceive life.

Think about this:

- You have been sorting through information about how things are, only to discover that your perceptions were often wrong.
- You have stored up untruths as truth.
- You are struggling with your issues of inadequacy and loving yourself.

Consequently, do you think you are the best person to define God? This question isn't meant to insult your intelligence or ability. It is to remind you that you have had so much distorted thinking in your life that your definition of God and your attitude about God have been adversely influenced.

This issue doesn't involve religion, sects, or denominations. It involves God. For now, I hope you'll accept a few statements about God, others, and yourself:

God is forgiveness.
God is love.
God cares.
God will never leave you or forsake you.
God is a loving God who allows mistakes to happen.
Every individual is a creation of God.

God accepts you as you.

You (and all persons) have worth because God made you.

God, and only God, is perfect and never fails

In the past few years we've heard stories about spiritual leaders who have led secret-but-sinful lives or who have gone astray. But that should not surprise us. All people, religious or not, fail.

The word *religion* may be a big turnoff to you because you have stored up misinformation as truth. Perhaps you got your "facts" from religious-but-unhealthy individuals.

I want to point you toward faith and love—the central messages of the God who created the human race. God's love tells us to do the right thing and then forgives us when we fail. I want you to experience a caring, healthy type of faith.

Find a church to meet that need. Don't put your faith in the people who belong to that particular church. If you have trouble with relationships, you'll see their faults and shortcomings and tend to cut yourself off from them. Stay with the group you choose until you can see them better. If they let you down, you're not going to give up on your faith in God. Put your faith in God and not in people because they will fail and God won't.

Remember this above everything else: You don't have to become adequate. You just have to be you. Then God will help you develop faith. God has already made you adequate, and you can learn to accept that reality.

Balance in your life is going to keep you from getting depressed, moody, angry, or frustrated over stressful situations. This concept of spirituality is a preventive approach. I want you to consider the spiritual damage that has gotten in the way so you can look forward to spiritual health.

EXERCISE 7:
ASSESSING SPIRITUAL DAMAGE

Let's look at where spiritual damage comes from. As you go through Exercise 7 and read an item that fits you, pause and say to yourself, "_____ (abuse issue) has created a conflict in the development of a healthy spiritual outlook." Mark the answers that apply to you.

1. Religious abuse

Have you been abused religiously? Have people in the past imposed their personal values on you by saying that's what God wants you to do? If that's the case and it's been done consistently, you may be suffering from religious abuse. That gets in the way of developing spirituality.

Religious Abuse Has Created a Conflict in the Development of a Healthy Spiritual Outlook: Yes ☐   No ☐

2. Emotional abuse

Perhaps you were put down, degraded, and made to feel insignificant as a child. If persons in authority spoke in ways that constantly made you feel not good enough or unacceptable, that was emotional abuse.

Emotional Abuse Has Created a Conflict in the Development of a Healthy Spiritual Outlook: Yes ☐   No ☐

3. Intellectual abuse

Frequently, people have been intellectually abused. They have been repeatedly called stupid, or else even their failures have been praised by others as being great.

Intellectual Abuse Has Created a Conflict in the Development of a Healthy Spiritual Outlook: Yes ☐   No ☐

4. Sexual abuse

Sexual abuse is very common, especially in alcoholic families. Did you experience sexual abuse at home or elsewhere?

Sexual Abuse Has Created a Conflict in the Development of a Healthy Spiritual Outlook: Yes ☐   No ☐

5. Parental abuse

Have you seen emotional problems with your parents? Were they angry people? Were they always throwing guilt at you?

Parental Abuse Has Created a Conflict in the Development of a Healthy Spiritual Outlook: Yes ☐   No ☐

If you answered yes to number five, put an X by the appropriate issues listed below.

_____ Socially. Did your parents drink, use drugs, or abuse food so that you related all that with social dynamics?

_____ Physically. Did your parents beat you, threaten to beat you, or physically abuse you in some other way? Did you fear being hurt? Were you afraid to make mistakes or to say the wrong thing because of past threats or abuse?

_____ Spiritually. Did your parents ignore the spiritual dimension, so they never talked about it? (Ignoring the spiritual dimension isn't normally considered abuse. But we consider ignoring a child's emotional needs a form of abuse. Neglecting such an integral part of a child as the spiritual being is as much an abuse.) Or did your parents deal with spirituality too much?

_____ Vocationally. Were your parents success oriented? Power oriented? Money oriented? Accomplishment oriented? Then you came second.

_____ Other issues. _____

These areas can create a conflict in the development of a healthy spiritual outlook. Share your results with your support person. You need to be able to look at options. Many of these issues may require outside help. Many of them are just a matter of recognizing that they exist and being able to deal with them.

TO CONFLICT OR NOT TO CONFLICT

Is it a conflict?

Let's define a conflict before you move into developing spiritual health. *Conflict* is a dilemma, a situation, a problem, an issue—something you confront that you have to resolve. Whether large or small, that is conflict. Unfortunately, you may be like many others who respond to things that are conflicts to you, but only because of your unrealistic expectations.

A few illustrations may help.

1. Helen says, "My son doesn't listen to me all the time. I talk, but he acts as if I'm not even in the room."

My answer: "Okay, your son doesn't listen all the time. I accept that as fact, but what's the conflict?"

"He doesn't listen—"

"That's not a conflict. Is it better to yell at him—which is conflict? Or is it better for you to accept a fact that your son just doesn't listen every time you speak?" That may not be right, but it is a correct statement, and it may be a more realistic expectation.

2. "My daughter doesn't do everything I ask her to." Is that, in itself, conflict? Or is it a conflict only if you expect her to do everything you ask?

3. "I didn't get all *A*'s on my report card." Is that a conflict because of an unrealistic expectation?

This may sound like a word game, but it isn't. First, you need to distinguish between fact and conflict. A situation becomes a conflict when you have standards that aren't met. Standards can be real, only perceived as legitimate, or unachievable.

Is it a conflict only for you?

Ask, Is this only *my* conflict? Am I the only one troubled or disturbed?

Often conflict is conflict because of your attitude. For example, all people pay taxes, but for whom does it create a conflict? For those who are burdened by the financial strain of taxes? For those who don't believe the government's use of their money is legitimate? Or for those who accept that taxes are a part of life and that government waste will always occur? Sometimes it is helpful to look at the total picture and see whether or not what is conflict to you is conflict to most people. It will help you determine whether or not you are overreacting or oversensitive to the issue because of some other need.

Why is it a conflict?

Why is having a disagreement with a spouse a conflict? Do we have to make an issue about which we disagree into a conflict?

What about the idea of having supper at a set time? Maybe you and your spouse disagree about that. Is that really a conflict? Or is that a conflict only for you? What is the big deal? Why do you have to have things your way?

Now you're getting to the real issue. Is the real issue a need for control? Is the real issue that you don't think your spouse listens to you? Or is the real issue that it gets in the way of something you want to do?

What is the real issue?

If the real issue is control, it won't matter what time you eat. Ask yourself, Am I being selfish? Am I trying to convince other people to do things my way so that I get my way? Am I having trouble with acceptance, unconditional love, and self-discipline? You create a conflict when you're being selfish.

What are your options?

"We can eat at five, six, or seven." You can compromise, or you can change. There are lots of options. You are never caught in a situation where no options exist.

A lot of people, for example, have said to me, "I don't have enough money, and I'm going to go broke."

I can offer them options. Here are a few:

- You can sell possessions you don't really need.
- You can drive one car and use public transportation.
- You can pack a lunch instead of spending six dollars every day for a noonday meal.
- You can buy less expensive clothes or wear what you have more often.

I can see an endless variety of options, but they seldom do. They are trying to do what they want and not take into account other options.

What happens if there are no solutions? (Occasionally, there are no solutions.) Even if there are options, sometimes the solution is too drastic or costly. What do you do then? It depends on the situation. If the conflict is with another person, you can say, "Here are my needs. I'd like to know yours." Then just step away from the situation, and you'll be amazed at the solution that can occur.

Often relationships end up with no solutions. Frequently, I see a wife (increasingly, husbands are saying this as well) who says, "I want more time with my spouse." The couple argue a lot. He insists his job saps all his free time and energy. They argue over priorities, money, free time, and every other subject. Each believes the other is wrong—and says so often. If he works less, however, they won't be able to keep up payments on the house. She wants to stay in their house. Quitting her dead-end job is no solution. It's then again a problem of finances.

This sounds like an impasse with no solution. However, there is no argument if she says (and means), "I want to spend more time with you because I love you, and I like being with you more than anyone else in the world."

He responds, "I would love to be with you, but I don't know how to spend time with you and hold down this job. I want to be with you." If this is true, again, there's no argument, although there is no solution.

If they can leave it and accept that there is no immediate solution, that they both have a problem, they can also realize that they will eventually find a way to resolve the dilemma— not now but soon.

Decide what you will do

Choose your course of action. By exercising self-discipline, you can do it.

THE SPIRITUAL REALM

After working with many people, I've come up with eight areas in the spiritual realm that cause the most difficulty.

1. Surrender to God

For many people, this concept is the most challenging to work with. Surrender to God embodies any of the following statements:

- "I am as totally open to God as I know how to be."
- "I turn to God because I trust that He cares and wants to guide me."
- "I am willing to rely on God, even though I don't understand what lies ahead."

• "I commit myself to God, and even though I don't understand, I don't have to keep trying to do everything my way."

I tell people who struggle with giving themselves up to God, "It is a process. It's like going to the beach to swim. Some people bravely jump in and take the plunge at once. You may have to begin by dipping your big toe into the water. Then you insert your whole foot. Take it slowly until your whole body is immersed. Whichever way works for you."

Control over your life may be so important to you that you don't want to give it up to anyone or anything. I hope you can perceive of God as One who loves you and wants only the best for you. If giving yourself is a big issue, start with the big toe in the water. You can start your surrender to God by saying, "God, this is as much as I am able to give. But I do give this much, and I want to trust You so that I can surrender more."

If that's honest, it's a prayer. It's also a way for you to begin to surrender to God.

2. Have unconditional love for yourself and for others

In the previous chapter we discussed this at length. I add only that you still have problems with unconditional love

• if you struggle with loving yourself and forgiving yourself regardless of your mistakes.

• if you struggle with loving and forgiving people around you when they make mistakes or don't do things your way.

3. Accept yourself and others

Can you really accept who you are? What you're not? What you are? When you honestly think of yourself and your abilities and achievements, can you do it without comparing yourself to the ideal or the ultimate?

Can you accept others? Do you feel people constantly let you down? Can you accept their imperfections and flaws and still see them as valuable human beings?

4. Be self-disciplined

Are you a person who decides to do something, goes at it for a while, and then stops? Do you get bored or find other things that interest you more? Do you start projects, but you can't seem to carry them through? No matter what excuse you make, self-discipline is a real issue for you if you do this regularly.

Earlier, I stressed the reward center and the importance of rewards. Your lack of self-discipline may mean that you have not set up a suitable payoff. You may do yourself the most good by looking again at your neurochemical profile and reconsidering your reward system.

5. Resolve spiritual conflicts

In Exercise 7 you assessed spiritual damage. Are there areas you haven't resolved? Are there issues or problems that prevent you from trusting a loving, caring, supportive God who forgives and accepts you as you are? Are you afraid to trust people because of your past experiences? Are you unable to get beyond your hurts and bruises?

These are all spiritual conflicts. Resolving them doesn't mean forgetting them. You'll never be totally free of them, but you don't stay with the same conflicts. As you grow, you encounter different issues or have clearer perceptions about your old ones. Resolving conflicts means that you are making progress. If the spiritual problems that once sent you into deep depression now cause you concern but you can move on, you are resolving your issues.

6. Listen more

As you've gone through this book and worked on your eating issues, has it occurred to you that you don't listen enough? Are you aware that you talk too much? Or even if you're not talking, you're not really hearing? Someone said, "We have to learn to listen with our hearts as well as our ears." He meant more than hearing words and processing information; we need to care about the persons who speak and their problems.

7. Share yourself

Have you discovered that you need to share more of yourself? In the past, you've defended your silence by saying, "I'm a very private person." Are you now beginning to consider that you may be too private? That you need to open up a little more of yourself to others?

8. Change your attitudes toward conflict

No one likes conflict. You may still see any conflict as a personal attack. When you become aware of conflict, do you ask yourself questions such as:

- Why is it a conflict?
- What's the *real* issue?
- Is this conflict only for me?
- Am I just being selfish?
- What are my options?
- What am I going to do that will be a healthy action?

Also ask yourself the following:

- Do I define life as "This is the way it's supposed to be..."?
- Do I get angry when things go wrong or don't go the way I planned?
- Do I hear myself saying things such as, "Why do other drivers always...?"

A "yes" answer to any of the last three questions indicates a negativity toward the conflicts of life. Work on developing a more positive attitude toward conflict.

EXERCISE 8:
DEVELOPING MY SPIRITUAL HEALTH

Put an X by the spiritual needs that you consider important in your growth toward and development of spiritual health. Fill in number nine if you think of other areas you need to concentrate on.

_____ 1. Surrender to God.
_____ 2. Develop unconditional love
     _____ a) for myself.
     _____ b) for others.

_____ 3. Develop full acceptance
      _____ a) of myself.
      _____ b) of others.
_____ 4. Develop self-discipline.
_____ 5. Resolve spiritual conflicts seen in Exercise 7.
_____ 6. Listen more to others.
_____ 7. Share more with others.
_____ 8. Change my attitude toward conflicts.
_____ 9. _____

When you have finished, review your list. Below, write the two issues that most concern you.

1. My most important issue is _____.
2. My second most important issue is _____.

Discuss the exercise with your support person. Ask,

- "Since you have been my support person, in which areas do you think I've already made progress?"
- "In which areas do you think I've made the most progress and in what way?"
- "From your knowledge of me, which two items would you have checked?"

After your discussion, you may wish to change your two items, or you may be convinced that these two are the most important.
The areas to which I commit myself toward developing my spiritual health are

1. _____.
2. _____.

22

— ♥ —

How I Appear to Others: My Personality Type

Consider the following statements.

- "I don't care what others think of me."
- "Other people's opinions of me don't matter. It's what I think of myself that counts."
- "I can't be bothered worrying about what anyone else thinks. It's like the song that says, 'I gotta be me.'"

These statements sound good. Unfortunately, they aren't true. We do care what others think of us because we are social creatures. We may discount or ignore their opinions, but they count. Remember when you lost weight and people commented? How did you feel? Remember when you wore clothing that got favorable attention? Wasn't it nice to be noticed?

Self-approval is important—more important—but the truth is, others mold us, shape our thoughts and attitudes. We need their input.

And it is true that "I gotta be me," but you don't become you in isolation. You become who you are in an environment. For example, you were raised in a home. Who you are today reflects that upbringing. You rigidly conformed to the home code, you blatantly rebelled, or (more likely) you did a little of both. But you used the opinions, attitudes, and values of others to shape and determine your own.

In your quest for recovery, you need outside validation. I've stressed throughout this book your need for a support system. Now you need others to recognize that you are different. You have changed.

Human nature is interesting. You know many things or sense them, but you need others to approve and endorse you. Let yourself think about the changes going on in your life. Doesn't it give you a good feeling and a stronger resolve when your friends make positive statements?

- "You're different. I like the changes I see in you."
- "You're quieter. Kinder, too, I think."
- "You've developed a real personality."
- "I liked you before; I like you a lot better now."

Especially if you're relationship oriented, it's going to be important for you to hear people say such things.

However, if no one notices or comments, it will be difficult for you to continue making changes. Of course, you will self-validate, no matter what. You'll be able to say to yourself, "I like who I'm becoming. I feel better about myself."

Another plus from outside validation is that words of affirmation and encouragement help you in your thought towers.

This leads up to the next step of looking honestly and objectively at how you appear to others. Denial may still be a problem for you. As you read the following personality types, your reaction may be, "Oh, sure, I'm a little like that, but I don't know if it's the problem. After all, it's not such a big deal."

This response implies denial. Before you fully change, you will have to be able to look honestly, even ruthlessly, at yourself and ask, Is this a picture of me?

FIVE PERSONALITY TYPES

I'm going to list five personality types. If you can see yourself in one or more of them, it's fair to say you are not alone. They are characteristic of others with food-dependency problems.

1. The Bear

Aggressive. Forceful. Intimidating. These words best describe the Bear personality.

Do you struggle with anger? A lot of frustration? A heavy load of stress that makes you erupt in anger or rage? Are you sometimes verbally or emotionally abusive? Do you put down others? Do you deny them compliments and praise when they deserve them?

Perhaps you've been physically abusive. This fact may be painful for you to face, but do it anyway if it describes you. You must face who you are so that you can change what you don't like in yourself. If you are or have been physically abusive, you need to look at your expectations and thought towers. You may need to seek professional help.

2. The Bunny

The Bunny is passive and avoids conflict. You may cross the street so you don't have to talk to someone. You run away from obstacles or hide from problems.

These may be some of your often-used expressions:

- "It's not my problem."
- "I don't want to deal with that now."
- "It's not that serious."

Do any of these sentences describe you? Your kids are screaming, your friends are in an uproar, but you are sitting and calmly observing it all. You shake your head at work-aholic students and think, *They just want to get the best grades*. You withdraw from things and detach yourself.

You may watch too much television. You sit in front of the TV and say little, but you snack, snack, snack. You think you ought to be interested in what's going on around you, but you're not.

If you are a Bunny, you tend to see yourself in the worst possible light. When you make a mistake, you use words such as *always* and *never*.

You may be saying these things to yourself or to others about yourself. (Each parenthetical statement is a better way to convey the message.)

- "I never do anything right."
  ("I didn't do it right this time, but I am learning to do better.")

• "I always say the wrong things."
　　("Sometimes I say the wrong things. I'm learn-
　　　ing to be more careful with my words.")

3. The Buffalo

Control, power, and self-assurance characterize Buffaloes. Buffaloes try to give the impression that a problem doesn't exist, they minimize its importance, or they say, "I've got it under control."

Do you work at convincing others that you have everything in your life under control? You say, "Eating isn't really a problem. I just like the taste of food. I'll go on a diet when I get too big." When conflicts arise, you say, "I'm in control here." Your spouse or friends complain, and you say, "Oh, yeah, I'll take care of it." Of course, you don't, but you give the impression that you'll handle it immediately.

Many Buffalo personalities are sexually addicted. Sex is a compelling, sometimes controlling force in their lives. They demand more sex from a single partner or from multiple partners. Or they could be what I call romance addicted—they want the opposite sex to think they are special and attractive.

4. The Bird

Passive-aggressive, withdrawn, smile-and-slap—the Bird doesn't do anything outwardly aggressive. It's the subtle put-down, the little jab at the end of a compliment: "She has turned out to be such a fine wife for my brother, especially considering what she was before he married her."

Or you may withdraw emotionally. You struggle between drawing close and distancing yourself. Can you recall times when you felt extremely close to someone and yet just as many times when you pulled back? At times, you seem open and approachable, and yet at other times, people seem to be afraid of you.

I watched a robin eat at our bird feeder one day. He pecked, jerked his head up and looked around, then bent his head down for another bite. A little later, the same robin perched on a branch. He sat unmoving until I was within ten feet. He showed no fear, no panic. Some personalities are like that—wary, suspicious, and yet sometimes open and trusting.

Do your friends ever comment that they have to figure out your mood? They say, "I'm not sure what you mean sometimes. Are you complimenting me or putting me down?"

You may even recognize that you have a problem, but you may feel that you're too busy to deal with it.

5. The Banshee

In Scottish folklore, a banshee is a female spirit who wails and warns of impending doom. The Banshee personality, therefore, is negative and complaining. For the Banshee, everything is a problem. I call it a life-is-an-if-only situation:

- "If only you would..."
- "If only the government would finally..."
- "If only the weather would..."
- "If only *they* would..."

The implication is that if things were different, you would be happy. Actually, you wouldn't. Even if they were different, you wouldn't be satisfied. You'd still be thinking how unfair life is. You are an "awfulizer" who keeps telling everyone how bad things are and they're getting worse:

- "Ain't life awful?"
- "Ain't it awful what they're doing in China?"
- "Ain't it awful what's going on in movies and videos these days?"
- "Ain't it awful the way people just don't care about anything anymore?"

If you're a Banshee, you may change jobs and friends regularly (or want to). You never seem to be without a serious problem. One time it's finances. The next time it's "this job is killing me." A few days later, you say, "If only I could get my kids straightened out."

You keep changing goals and problems, never seeing anything as your fault. It's always "them" or "they" or the government or your ex-husband or the economic system.

EXERCISE 9:
BASIC PERSONALITY TYPE

1. Now that you have read the five descriptions, decide which one (or combination) *you* think best describes you. Put an X in the space.

Of the five, the description that fits me is

____ A Bear.
____ A Bunny.
____ A Buffalo.
____ A Bird.
____ A Banshee.

I also see that I am a combination of _____

_____.

2. You are ready to commit yourself to change. Here is your self-affirmation.

———————— ♥ ♥ ♥ ————————

Vital facts about myself: I see changes in my life. I like who I am becoming.

———————— ♥ ♥ ♥ ————————

3. Show your response to your support person. Ask the following questions:

- "In what ways do you think I have perceived myself accurately?"
- "In what ways do you think I have perceived myself inaccurately?"
- "What positive changes have you recognized in me since I started my self-recovery program?"

4. If you're comfortable enough, go to your spouse, a family member, or someone else you feel close to, and explain about the basic personality types. Ask,

- "Which of these descriptions do you think fits me?"
- "Which do you think fits you?"

You may want to ask the questions you asked your support person.

I suggest going to another person because everybody is a combination of strengths and weaknesses. You need to see your strengths and weaknesses. It also helps you to see them in others, especially those who can honestly accept both their strengths and weaknesses.

Once you feel confident that you've accurately identified your personality type, you are ready to examine your communication style. Your communication style is the second major factor in how you appear to others.

23

♥

How I Appear to Others: My Communication Style

You may feel you don't get enough support. If people were more supportive or supportive in a different way, things would be better. Then you'd feel much more comfortable.

In the previous chapter I asked you to look at the addictive characteristics of your personality type. Even when you can admit these traits, it will take courage and commitment for you to deal with them.

But before you start to work on these personality traits, please understand, you are *not* a Bear, Bunny, Buffalo, Bird, or Banshee. These are shorthand terms to help you see your problem areas. They express something about you, but the term you chose doesn't apply to who you are.

Here is the most significant self-affirmation you can make about yourself.

───────── ♥ ♥ ♥ ─────────

Vital facts about myself: I am a lovable, worthwhile child of God. God loves me and accepts me as I am; I love and accept myself as I am.

───────── ♥ ♥ ♥ ─────────

COMMUNICATION STYLES

Although I want you to see the positive side of yourself, the way you appear to others may prevent them from supporting you. Quite likely the first way they got to know you was through your communication style. My use of the word *communication* includes the way you use every part of yourself—your voice, body, gestures, posture, and mood. I stress how others perceive you for one basic reason: If others don't know you, they can't help much.

Understanding how you appear to others can help you better understand why you sometimes get supported and why you don't at other times. You can then begin to figure out how you can make changes to gain better support.

1. "You need to do it this way"

Maybe you know Controlling Cathy. If you're like her, you're good at telling others what to do and how to do it. When people start talking about problems, you say, "Now this is what you want to do..." However, if they don't do it, you get angry or disgusted with them.

If this sounds like you, it is difficult for you to get the kind of support you need because you want to control the support person.

Your controlling may be a defensive action. That is, if you keep the power in your hands, you set the limits of the conversation with your support person. Although you do it unconsciously, you keep control by

- changing the subject when the person gets too close.
- inserting jokes or humor to lessen your anxiety.
- focusing on a minor issue instead of a major one.

2. "I know exactly"

Power Pete frequently says, "I know." He is different from Controlling Cathy, who is committed to dominate and decide for others, because he is more concerned about himself. Power Pete uses power to resist self-change.

If you're related to Power Pete, you may be tagged as a know-it-all. You have the answer to everything. If that fits you, I want you to do a little backtracking. Try to think of situations where you said,

- "I don't know."
- "That's not my area of expertise."
- "I don't have an opinion on that topic."

Being unable to readily think of saying such a thing may indicate your need for power. Power is the opposite of helplessness. Often people who felt helpless as children, especially in dysfunctional families, overcompensate by grabbing for power. Feeling helpless and unprotected may be the worst thing you can think of.

3. "That's the way"

Are you a Dismissive Donna? Does this happen in your home? Your kids come to you and say, "Look at this! I did this."

"That's just fine," you say, "and now, I want you to try..."

You have taken the compliment that affirmed their accomplishment ("That's just fine") and blown it apart because you wanted more ("And now..."). You gave the compliment with one breath and took it away with the next. You dismissed their effort as unimportant. Your agenda was more important.

Here's another example. In second grade, Tim colored a picture. He was especially proud of the color choices of the leaves. As soon as his dad walked into the house, he rushed at him with the picture. He said, "See, Dad! I did this in school. Isn't this neat?"

"Yeah, that's really great." Dad looked over the picture. "Next time, do it a little more carefully. Be sure not to go outside the lines. See?" He pointed to the "mistake."

What did Dad really say? "Tim, I don't like your picture because you colored outside the lines."

That's a negative communication style. Do you tend to respond that way?

4. "That's fine, but..."

Does But Barry sound like you? You intend to compliment. You want to say something nice, but you also feel you have to be honest—or so you tell yourself. You offer the compliment but quickly tack on a criticism: "Say, you did a great job mowing the lawn, but you missed a spot near the mailbox."

This style is close to "That's the way." The difference here is that you call it constructive criticism. You are teaching and showing a better way to do things. When you pass on a compliment, you can't resist putting a little twist at the end.

- To your wife: "Honey, you're a good cook...compared to your sister."
- To your husband: "You're thoughtful, especially when I compare you to the man I almost married."
- To your child: "That's pretty good for you."
- To a coworker: "You did a good job, especially for someone without a college degree."

5. "I should have..."

Does Shoulda Sally's style fit you? She is a wonderful second-guesser. She knows the right decision and will tell you gladly—especially after you have already made the wrong one.

A friend told me about this incident from his boyhood. He was playing with a bullet for a .22 rifle. He ground down the point and put it on the sidewalk. With a hammer he struck the bullet so that it fired. Unfortunately, part of the shell went into his leg. He not only felt the pain, but the blood streaming down caused him to panic. He screamed and started toward the house.

Just then his father came running out to him. As soon as he realized what had happened, the father said, "You should have been more careful. If you had been, you wouldn't have had this accident." As far as my friend was concerned, his dad didn't recognize his pain. The boy interpreted this and other similar statements from his father to mean that he was never right and that he always made the wrong choices.

If you have a Shoulda Sally communication style, you say things such as,

- "I should have married someone else."
- "I should have gone to a different school."
- "I should have changed jobs a year ago."

The shoulda types live in regret. They know the right choice only after they have made a wrong one.

6. "That's fine...just fine"

For Plastic Paul, everything is fine. No one is wrong. Everyone is fine, lovely, sweet, kind, and thoughtful. If two people are having an argument, Plastic Paul smiles at both of them. Afterward, he says to each in private, "You were right."

If you're like Plastic Paul, no one really knows you or your values. Some may think of you as an individual with no depth. In reality, you don't want to hurt anyone. You're everybody's friend—except you don't have any friends. You can never be a real friend until the other person knows who you are.

7. "That was dumb and it was terrible"

Critical Clara is more direct than most communicators. She excuses her approach with statements such as,

- "That's just the way I am."
- "I'm just an honest person."
- "I calls 'em as I sees 'em."
- "If you don't like hearing the truth, just don't ask me anything."
- "If I criticize you, it's only because I want the best for you."

If you're like Critical Clara, criticism is a major part of your personality. But you don't use the word *criticism*; you speak of your candor or your sense of integrity. Being honest equals being critical. You also think that giving compliments makes others lazy and indifferent and destroys their incentive.

You think that if you point out failings and shortcomings of others, you're motivating them to change. Actually, it's better to praise people for what they've done and encourage them instead of criticizing them for what they *haven't* done.

8. "Did you know...?"

Gossiping Gus spreads the news quickly, not always accurately, and sometimes maliciously. And, yes, I know that a large part of our population gossips. One reason, I believe, is that speaking or spreading bad news about others is a way to make you feel smug and superior—momentarily anyway.

If you don't think of yourself as Gossiping Gus, are you his twin brother Listening Lenny? He listens to all the gossip. He makes no effort to stop it, even if he doesn't pass it on. If you are Gossiping Gus or Listening Lenny, stop and consider that gossip does you no good. It doesn't build up anyone or change anything positively.

I was amazed a few years ago to realize how much the Bible speaks against bearing tales and spreading gossip. It's a harmful practice, and it's self-destructive because it makes you think in negative categories. Gossip clogs your mind with stories of failures and shortcomings. If you want to change, you'll spend no time with Gossiping Gus and Listening Lenny.

9. "How could you?"

This line is a favorite of Guilt-Giver Gertie. Here are some of her most famous sayings:

- "It was wrong to do it that way."
- "You weren't raised to ..."
- "I went to all that trouble to make that meal special for you. Now you don't want it."
- "But, darling, you always like cheese in your casserole. I mean, I bought it special ..."
- "Now the Bible says ..."

The last one is a powerful tool of Guilt-Giver Gertie because she uses it not to give information but to condemn and prove others wrong. "Once they know they are wrong and sinful, they'll have to face up to their sins," she says in defense, never asking who ordained her to pronounce the sentence of guilt.

Guilt is a real killer. If you're a friend of Guilt-Giver Gertie, you probably had guilt used on you. That's how you learned to do it effectively. But you also know how it hurts you and how much you'd like to get the guilt giver out of your life.

EXERCISE 10:
YOUR COMMUNICATION STYLE

Read each of the communication styles. As you read, ask yourself, Is this how I appear to others? You need to face these parts of yourself. But remember that you face them so you can change; you can become more positive, more caring, and more open. Once you move in that direction, you'll also realize that people respond differently to you. You're likely to feel that your needs are being met more effectively. You'll feel you have traveled a long way down the road of resolving many of your conflicts and stresses.

You may feel you fit in several categories. Select the two that you think describe you best. Put an X by those two.

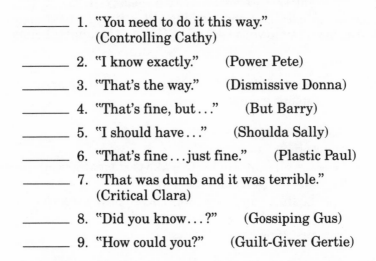

1. "You need to do it this way."
   (Controlling Cathy)

2. "I know exactly."   (Power Pete)

3. "That's the way."   (Dismissive Donna)

4. "That's fine, but..."   (But Barry)

5. "I should have..."   (Shoulda Sally)

6. "That's fine...just fine."   (Plastic Paul)

7. "That was dumb and it was terrible."
   (Critical Clara)

8. "Did you know...?"   (Gossiping Gus)

9. "How could you?"   (Guilt-Giver Gertie)

After you have gone through this exercise, show your two responses to your support person. Ask your support person the following questions:

- "In what ways do you think I have perceived myself accurately?"
- "In what ways do you think I have perceived myself inaccurately?"
- "What positive changes have you recognized in me since I started my self-recovery program?"

If you're comfortable enough, go to your spouse, a family member, or someone else you feel close to, and explain that you are concerned about how the person perceives you. Ask,

- "Which of these descriptions do you think fits me?"
- "Which do you think fits you?"

You may also want to ask the same questions you asked your support person. You will begin to get an idea of your actual communication styles. And you will be able to begin changing those styles that keep others from supporting you.

24

— ♥ —

Approaching Life

Whenever the news media inform us of a mass killing or the capture of a serial murderer, they interview neighbors and co-workers of the offender. In almost every instance, the people interviewed say something like this: "Why, he was so kind. Never gave anyone any trouble."

The criminals are not known as they really are—their public side contrasts sharply with their private side.

Reflect on yourself right now and how others think of you. The public you—the part that interacts with other human beings—is that the same person as the private you?

Who are you? How do you approach life? Do you like to be quiet? Are you laid-back and willing to go with the flow? Do you keep things to yourself? Are you known for your openness? "What you see is exactly who I am," said one gregarious friend.

There are any number of ways you can define yourself. Are you someone who likes to paint with a broad brush? Or would you rather do detail work? Do you insist on a logical flow from one idea to another? Are you more intuitive so that you come up with right answers, but you don't know what process you used to get there? Do you approach life from an emotional viewpoint or an intellectual one? Do you see things first from the heart or from the head? Are you a structured person who wants to know when to start and when to finish? Do you make out lists and follow them?

Knowing who you are—in your inmost self—is fundamental

to your recovery. There are no bad approaches to life. You are simply different from every other person in the world. All are acceptable ways to approach life. The more fully you know who you are, the more easily you can cope with your conflicts.

I've set up an exercise to help you recognize how you approach life.

EXERCISE 11:
BASIC APPROACHES TO LIFE

After you read each explanation, make a choice. Think in terms of your *preferred* attitude. Put an X by the choice that describes you.

Public or Private?

The private person tends to be more introspective. If you look inward for answers, this probably speaks of you.

If you like being with people and feel energized in their presence, you are a public person.

The private tends not to want to share experiences, while the public is often eager to do so.

_____ I am private.

_____ I am public.

Detailer or Generalist?

"Just give me the main idea," says the generalist. The detailer wants to know every fact, important or not.

Do you like to collect as much information as possible and then come up with a solution? Or do you prefer to grasp the concept and work from that?

A generalist is often the idea person, the one who speaks in terms of the what, the idea, and the concept. A detailer asks questions such as, "How? When? Why?"

_____ I am a detailer.

_____ I am a generalist.

Emotional or Intellectual?

Do you tend to make decisions based on feelings, or do you weigh negatives against positives before choosing? Do you like things that are intellectually stimulating, or do you like things that are more emotionally oriented?

_____ I am emotional.

_____ I am intellectual.

Structured or Unstructured?

Do you make lists of your activities to do each day? Maybe you even have an A list for top priority, a B list to turn to next, and a C list for any free time? Or do you like to take life as it comes? That is, do you say, "I like to wing it"?

Of course, some people work in highly structured jobs and adapt well. Yet, by preference, they are more flexible and fluid in their attitudes. An example is someone who works all day with exacting information but at home enjoys lying on the sofa and watching television.

_____ I am structured.

_____ I am unstructured.

You now have your basic approach to life. Do the following things with your responses to Exercise 11.

1. Show the responses to your support person. Sometimes people react to what they want to be or think they should be instead of what they are. Ask your support person to evaluate your answers. You may need to rethink one or more of them.

2. "We just seem to have one hassle after another." About whom do you make this statement? Is it your spouse, best friend, child, parent, or supervisor? Once you select the individual(s), you may choose to pursue any of the suggestions that follow. Bear in mind that the exercise is not to change the other person or yourself. It is not to fix anything. The purpose is to see that you approach life differently. You may discuss ways each can learn to accept and accommodate the other.

• Set aside some time to meet with that person and show your results. (Meet with more than one person if necessary.)

• Share where you see yourself, and let the person see the differences between you. Sometimes simply rec-

ognizing the distinctions makes relationships easier for both parties.

- On your own, go through the four approaches of
these significant people. Try to see where you are
similar and where you are different. You'll likely
discover that the conflicts lie within a certain area,
such as one being structured and the other unstructured.

Your approaches *are* different. That's the point of the exercise. If you're a detailer and your son is a generalist, you may
view him as a dreamer. He may see you as a person who
destroys dreams or has no imagination and you get bogged
down in details. If you're an intellectual man, your wife may
think you are unfeeling and unromantic. You may think of her
as somewhat flighty, highly overcharged with emotions.

Again I stress that neither is wrong. It is just the basic
approach to life. You must grasp this idea to be able to overcome your tendency to criticize and judge those who are
different.

If you are like most people, you think about what you
believe and value. Because you have thought it through, you
see this as truth. The tendency is to believe your "truth" is the
only truth. Because you see life one way, that is the only way to
see life. But if you can say something like the following, you
can begin to overcome your hassles: "Wait a minute! It's not a
matter of right or wrong. We just don't have the same approach
to life."

I want to share an example of how this works. A couple in
their late sixties are true pillars of their church. They give
generously and serve others in dozens of ways. They are probably the best-loved couple in the congregation. Yet one day the
wife was complaining, "These younger folks joining the church
don't seem to have a real commitment to God."

Her husband answered, "Or is it that their commitments
are different from ours?" After he saw a puzzled look on her
face, he said, "Honey, you and I grew up in a different era. The
church was the center of our lives, and we were taught that
everything revolved around that building and the people. They
come from a different era with different values."

"You know," she said, "I never thought of that before."

If you can accept that you approach life differently from other people, you are well on your way to resolving many of your conflicts.

♥ ♥ ♥

Vital facts about myself: I acknowledge that I have an approach to life that is my own. All people do not have the same approach.

♥ ♥ ♥

25

— ♥ —

Communication Changes

Obviously, improving communication skills is important, especially if you want to be more supportive of others. As you become more supportive, people tend to become more positive toward you. The following exercise can help you make changes that will allow for and improve communication.

EXERCISE 12:
BASIC WAYS TO ENHANCE
MY PERSONALITY

As you read an item and you say, "I need to work on that," put an X next to the number. When you finish, you will have a list of issues you can examine and think about as you seek to improve the way people see you.

_____ 1. I will be less negative. Are you negative? Do you look at just the worst? Do you focus on what people aren't? If so, you need to look at more of the positive things in life.

Seeing yourself as you *are* is more important than seeing yourself the way you want to be. So be honest with yourself. If you are now a negative person, you're not less of a person. You know a weakness, and you are ready to do something to change.

_____ 2. I will be less opinionated. Are you a Bear, a Buffalo, or a Banshee? Do you always have to offer an opinion on everything? You may find that people hesitate to share deeply with you because you're constantly giving them advice, regardless of whether they ask for it.

_____ 3. I will be more complimentary. Think about the number of times

- you say to your parents,
  "I appreciate the way you've tried to raise me."
- you say to your kids,
  "I appreciate you. You're neat."
- you say to your spouse,
  "You mean a lot to me. You've made my life so much better."
- you say to your friend,
  "Thank you for being my friend. It means a lot to me to know that you're with me."

Nobody gets enough compliments; nobody gives enough. As long as they are genuine, they can enrich and encourage others immensely.

_____ 4. I will share my needs more openly. Do you need to open up more? Do you cheat the important people in your life out of the opportunity to care for you when you're hurt or confused?

If you take an intellectual approach to life, you don't have to learn to share your inner self with everybody. But you do need to commit yourself to learning to open up appropriately. Select a friend, your support person, or your spouse to share your frustrations with.

_____ 5. I will be more supportive of others. You may declare that _you_ need more support. But if you feel you need more support, one of the best ways to get it is to be more supportive of others. It's a rule of life: If you give more, you'll receive more.

Being supportive doesn't mean that you must understand everything and approve of everything persons say and do.

Two examples may make this clear. First, Rob was forty-seven when he first began to deal with a childhood of physical and sexual abuse. He started to open up to his wife who had come from a sheltered background. "Rob, I don't understand what's going on inside you," she said, "but I'm here, and I'm with you all the way." Five years later, he said to me, "Her support gave me the courage to work on those childhood issues."

Second, Lyn's teenage daughter slowly became rebellious, refused to attend church, and threatened to leave home. "Do whatever you have to do," Lyn said, her eyes filled with tears. "But whatever you decide, I want you to know that I will never stop caring about you."

The daughter did leave. It took years for her to get straightened out. At her worst she was a topless dancer. When a friend found out, he asked, "What does your mother think of the way you live?"

The daughter said, "She may not like it, but she loves me."

Being supportive says, "I may not understand, but I believe in you, and I stand with you no matter what."

_____ 6. I will work fewer hours. Decide on a limit and say, "I will work thirty-eight hours each week." If you're a workaholic, you especially need to think about making this commitment.

_____ 7. I will work more faithfully. I will work a full week's hours. If you're lazy or tend to spend time on the job doing things for yourself such as making personal calls, you may need to look at this closely.

_____ 8. I will watch less TV. Say, "I will watch only _____ hours each week."

TV is a real communication blocker. It stops people from spending time talking to each other. Or they limit their conversations to the commercial breaks. Or they talk, but at least half their attention is on the TV set.

_____ 9. I will spend more time with my family. If you're a kid, how much time do you spend with your family? Are you busy trying to spend time away from them because they're no fun? What if you did something together?

If you're a parent, how much time do you actually spend with the family? Don't excuse yourself with the bit about working hard to make a decent livelihood for them. They need you more than they need things.

_____ 10. I will plan fun weekly activities with my friends/ family. What about planning more activities? Do you need to do things more with the family, with friends, with your spouse? Do you need to set aside date nights? Do you need to have those talks about some of those things?

_____ 11. I will spend more time (or less time) with my friends. Friends are the people who are not related to you, but they are there for you because they care. They need you, and you need them.

You can spend too much time with friends, especially if your approach to life is to be public oriented. You may need to cut back. But if you're private oriented, it may be time for you to say, "I want to enjoy my friends, and I do that by spending time with them."

_____ 12. I will exercise regularly. You may ask, "How can exercising improve my communication skills?" When you're frustrated, a workout, a fast-paced walk, or aerobics can alter your thoughts and decrease your negative emotions.

If you commit yourself to an exercise program and stay with it, you will feel better about yourself. (Of course, you need to choose the exercise that's right for you—as I showed you in chapter 14.)

_____ 13. I will follow my eating plan. Do you need to eat better? Watch your diet? Be more consistent? Are you a bear when you're hungry? When you haven't eaten right, do you get grumpy? Moody? How you eat determines how you feel.

_____ 14. I will set up and keep a daily quiet appointment with myself. Do you have time to sit down and look at who you really are? To backtrack and think about your progress? If you're public oriented, this step may be difficult for you, but it can be immensely beneficial.

Are you so busy keeping up that you don't even know where you've been or where you're running?

I recall a story about a young man who went to a wise old man. The young man said, "You know, sir, I'd like to be the best master in the world. I understand you're the best, so I've come here."

"That's really an ambitious undertaking. How much time are you going to put into it?"

"I'll work at this every day of my entire life, every waking minute I'll work at being a master and understanding people," the young man said. "But how long would it take me?"

"About thirty years."

"That's a long time," the young man said. Then he started to think about every day of his life seven days a week for thirty years. He didn't know if he could do it. So he asked, "What if I spent only about forty hours a week doing it? And taking weekends and evenings off?"

"Maybe twenty-five years."

The answer confused the young man. "But that means it takes less time."

"That is correct."

"Hmmm," the young man said. "What if I just check in every once in a while on how I'm doing, while I go on with life, work on my own. How long then?"

"Well, it may take you twenty years."

Now thoroughly confused, the young man said, "I don't understand. You say that working on myself and focusing on myself all the time, virtually every minute of every day, will take thirty years? But if I do other things and work on myself just now and then, it will take only twenty? Why the difference?"

The old man peered into the young man's eyes: "You know when you have both eyes looking to the future, trying to see what you're going to be, you'll amble off the path and wander around a lot. But if you keep one eye on the path of where you are and the other eye on where you want to be, it will take you a whole lot less time."

This old story illustrates essentially what I mean. Set up short periods of daily time out from your hectic schedule. Take time to find out whether you're running for a dream or whether you're on the path.

Here are suggestions for your private time:

- Keep a journal and record your thoughts and feelings.
- Draw yourself daily pictures of your mood and sense of being.
- Use a question-and-answer format in a journal. (Example: How do you see you are making progress? How do you feel about yourself today?)

_____ 15. I will attend a worship service regularly. You meet people who are concerned about the spiritual parts of their lives. No group of people is perfect, but you can find a congregation where you feel comfortable if you search for one.

_____ 16. I will pray daily. Do you need to pray more? Do you need to talk to God to gain insights? Many people don't understand prayer. If you try to figure out your issues totally on your own, you will have a difficult time because you don't see life realistically. That's why you enlist support people. That's also why you pray.

A word from the book of Proverbs applies here:

Trust in the LORD with all your heart. Never rely on what you think you know. Remember the LORD in everything you do, and he will show you the right way. Never let yourself think that you are wiser than you are; simply obey the LORD and refuse to do wrong. If you do, it will be like good medicine, healing your wounds and easing your pains (Prov. 3:5–8 TEV).

_____ 17. I will study the Bible every day. The Bible is the ultimate word of truth. Aside from that, the Bible is filled with words of wisdom and guidance. You can also learn from the examples and mistakes of other men and women of the past.

_____ 18. If you are aware of issues you need to change and to commit yourself to, write them here. I will _____

_____

_____.

Record the four most important issues from Exercise 12: Basic Ways to Enhance My Personality. Note that I used the word *enhance* in the title. Changing personalities is difficult; enhancing isn't.

You're going to be looking at how people interact with you and how you interact with yourself. But you need to honestly view how other people perceive you.

If you look at the personality types and communication types, you'll find out there are reasons why people are afraid of you or don't support you. There are reasons why you need support and you don't get it. You're not going to change others so they'll want to support you. You're not going to alter your personality drastically. You can change somewhat, and you can soften up. As this happens to you, you make yourself easier for people to support.

Go through this exercise with your support person and someone else close to you. Choose someone whose support you need. Say, "I want to share something with you—an exercise I've been working on. I want to try to figure out how I am to you. Please don't criticize me or tell me everything I ought to do. Just listen and give me your honest opinion."

When you speak this way, you have set the guidelines. They won't help you if they criticize. But they can help you if they say something such as, "Yeah, you know, sometimes you are a little on the aggressive side."

Don't try to fix yourself. Hear the responses. At this point, you're trying to figure out how others perceive you. Once you learn that, you can then figure out how to get validation. As you listen, you can grow. Your openness in asking others to listen to you is a big step in being validated and supported.

♥ ♥ ♥

Vital facts about myself:

I am a growing, changing person. I like the person I am becoming.

♥ ♥ ♥

26

♥

Your Emotional Issues

When you overeat, your emotions change. If you continue to overeat, you set up the changed emotion to be permanent. You store the information inside your brain that says how you feel when you overeat. Because you changed the emotion with a substance (food, but it could have been drugs or some form of behavior), your brain took this in as the new norm for you. Because it becomes normal when it is really abnormal, you can see how it easily affects your viewpoint and your reasoning.

Here are three scenarios. Maybe one sounds something like you.

1. You used to make presentations at work. You knew your material because you had been working on it for weeks. You spoke with self-confidence. Your brain stored this as a normal event.

For the past few months, however, you have been abusing food, you've got more and more tension in your life, and you have a feeling that your supervisor wants you to fail. Now what happens? Over a period of time, the combination of food and stress has intervened. When you're asked to do a presentation, you say, "Oh, no! I don't want to do it." You might even add, "I'm not good at making presentations." Your self-confidence level is down. Your brain chemicals have changed and stored new data that say, "I am not good at making presentations."

Although you're the same person, in many ways you have changed. In just this area where you used to do an excellent job, you now feel insecure. You avoid the task. You're afraid. Your emotions get all tied up when you think about the presentation.

2. Before food became a significant part of your life, you recall that you were able to sit and talk for long periods. You held your children on your lap. You liked to communicate with your spouse and close friends. If you were dating, you could talk endlessly, or so it seemed.

You might never have made any connection, but after a disastrous relationship, you felt rejected and unloved. You turned to food to find comfort and to take away your pain. You slowly changed.

Now you hate long conversations. You don't want to tell others about yourself or how you're feeling. When people try to talk to you, you're suspicious. Just the other day, a coworker invited you to lunch. You asked yourself, What does he want from me? Five years ago you wouldn't have had such a thought. The situation is much the same as before, but you are now processing the information differently. Your emotional response is different, too.

3. You come from what is now being termed a *dysfunctional family system*. The kindest way to put it is that your parents didn't get along. Your mother screamed at your dad. Sometimes she threw dishes or other things at him. When she punished you, she beat you with a belt. Your dad, however, was passive. He showed no emotion. He sometimes said, "I just want a little peace around here."

Emotional issues charged through the house. You hated your childhood. Stuffing yourself with food was the only way you got away from the noise and the upheaval. While you were still a child, those things began to affect your emotions.

You're married, and your husband says, "I wish you could just be a little supportive of me. I wish you could feel something." His words surprise you. You think you are supportive, and you don't know what he means.

Because of your dysfunctional family system, you're probably also what we now refer to as *codependent*. The common definition is that you can't find or don't find happiness in yourself. You look to someone else or depend on another person to make you happy. (In my book *Help Yourself,* you can find more information about codependency and these dynamics.)

I've described three situations, but there are thousands of ways of presenting emotional issues. Each of them is trying to make three points: (1) you used food as a way to escape your pain or discomfort or unhappiness; (2) the prolonged situations changed your neurochemistry, which means that your emotions have been affected; and (3) you probably aren't aware of this change, and you can't understand why you feel the way you do.

Previously, I pointed out the source of emotions—a result of spiritual conflict. You looked at surrendering to God and issues such as acceptance, unconditional love, and self-discipline. These conflicts bring about some thoughts in your thought tower. Your thought kicks in a neurochemical change. Out of the neurochemical change comes a different emotion.

For you, the neurochemical changes came about because of your food dependency. You changed emotionally without even being aware. Out of the emotional change you might have developed physical effects such as ulcers, high blood pressure, or headaches. Neurochemical changes can cause psychological changes such as depression and anxiety. Or they might have affected you spiritually, and your relationship with God deadened. Your view of life is confused and negative. You have difficulty perceiving reality clearly, or you have a strong denial system.

In this chapter, I want you to focus on the emotional part of yourself. You can begin to live differently. Learning to live differently will make you feel better about who you are, but it will also gain you validation from others. They will begin to perceive you differently because you will be different.

Let's delve into some common emotional issues of individuals who have been using food to deal with troublesome situations. I've observed these issues while working with hundreds of food-dependent persons. As you read through this material, I hope you'll be able to say, "Yes! That's exactly what I've experienced." After you stop overeating, these issues will eventually diminish, and you can get to the real issues in your life.

DENIAL

You experience this common emotion even if at times you say, "I wish I could control the amount of food I eat. I really want to stop overeating."

You have a problem. You know it. But you may not know the significance of the problem. Typically within your own system, your brain chemistry and your psychological system decide that you have to protect yourself. That's what denial does.

Your brain starts to interpret. (I don't agree with the viewpoint that food chemical dependency is only a weakness.) You just don't want to admit any shortcoming or problem to yourself. It's as if you say to your brain, "I don't want to face the fact that I have to cut my eating in half. I don't want to admit that I'm filled with rage and resentment." Your brain comes to your aid! "No problem. I'll just help you deny it."

Your brain and your unconscious "scheme" to protect you from harsh reality by creating the denial process, which enables you to say to yourself and others:

- "I really don't have that problem."
- "I can handle this. No big deal."
- "Other people have the same problem or worse, so what's the noise about?"
- "Oh, sure, I eat too much sometimes, but I like the taste of food."

The denial system also kicks in when you look at what your dependency is *not* doing to you. You say things such as, "You say it's a problem, and maybe it is for some, but it doesn't affect my work." Or you can insert words such as *family, competence,* or *relationships*. Your denial has focused on what you are able to do while you do something negative. You're saying, "I don't have the problem because I can still do these things, and it's not affecting this part of my life."

That may be true. But your food dependency has taken away your ability to mature and to move forward in your inner life.

You'll probably have a certain amount of denial. You may minimize the problem, insisting, "Well, I'm not all that bad." This attitude is a protective device that keeps you from seeing reality. You don't have to break your denial system down totally, but you need to understand that it plays games with you. That's the purpose of denial.

SELF-PROTECTION OR DEFENSIVENESS

When somebody says, "I really care for you, and I think that you have a problem," self-protection rushes in and pushes your denial system to say, "I don't really have a problem." Then you get defensive. You may attack:

- "Just who do you think you are to say that?"
- "Are you little Miss Perfect herself?"
- "Listen, clean up the mess in your own life before you try to straighten out somebody else."

At work you make a serious mistake. Your supervisor says, "You didn't do that right."

You respond, "Well, nobody explained it to me." Or you say, "There was so much noise in this place, I'm surprised I could do anything right."

Defensiveness rushes into the foray because you're trying to protect yourself from attack of any kind. You don't want anyone to see your imperfections. You don't want to hear that you are food dependent. You don't want to hear anything that you can't readily absorb.

Self-protection is an automatic reaction to attack. It is one of those responses to the ringing of the bell. Remember the process: You have a thought that raises up an internal conflict that leads to a feeling (emotion) that leads to a chemical change that leads to a new emotion that results in action. The bell goes off at the moment of thought. Since the bell has already gone off, it's difficult for you to perceive that you have shifted into a defensive mode.

Suppose your mother says, "You know, when you were young, you were warm and loving and caring. Why can't you be like that sweet child?"

You immediately state, "You're the one who has changed. You're not very caring anymore." Or you say, "Anyone who has had to go through the hard knocks I've gone through couldn't help changing." That is a defensive reaction. You are protecting yourself from assault or from emotional injury.

HOPELESSNESS

I don't know if you've tried to work on your problem with overeating before. You might have gone to a treatment center, been in an outpatient program, or tried to take care of your eating problem on your own.

No matter what way you've gone in the past, quite likely a voice in the back of your head whispers, "You can't do it." After all, you've read statistics that show it's difficult to make the kind of changes that will last all your life. Or one of your so-called friends says, "I've never seen anyone who got her weight under control and kept it that way. Sure enough, they all slip up if you give them time." You listen to those voices, and a sense of hopelessness comes over you.

Because many of the programs didn't try to fit an individual's personality, they didn't work. Everyone with a food-related problem isn't the same as five thousand others. But *The Help Yourself Love Yourself Nondiet Weight Loss Plan* aims to help you help yourself by fitting your program to your unique personality.

We tend to think not of uniqueness but of sameness. Consider what happened with penicillin. Newly discovered penicillin was hailed as the wonder drug, the one drug that cured everyone's infections. It was the antibiotic drug that worked. You know what happened? Some people went to a doctor with a simple infection, got an injection of penicillin, and became deathly ill. A few actually died. All of those individuals had allergic reactions. Most people can and do get splendid results from penicillin, but it's not for everyone.

The same mentality was at work in the field of chemical dependency—and still is in some areas. We gave it a nice term like *addictive personality*, which meant that the disease was the same for everyone, even though the drugs used were different. If the cause was the same, obviously the cure would be the same. The most commonly used treatment involved counseling and twelve-step programs patterned after Alcoholics Anonymous. The programs worked. That is, they worked for the people who tried them and stayed with them.

What can we say about the people who didn't make it through a twelve-step program? What was wrong? The experts said to them:

- "You're denying your problem."
- "You have to hit bottom—reach the place of utter desperation—first."
- "You say you want to be cured, but you just aren't ready."
- "If you would really commit yourself, you could do it."

Since the cure-all didn't cure all, obviously the sick ones were wrong. Or so the logic has said, and the nonachievers felt even more hopeless than before.

The Help Yourself Love Yourself Nondiet Weight Loss Plan provides a highly individualized plan. You don't have to live with the feeling of hopelessness. You can find ways to press the right buttons that open the doors for you to get free. I believe you want complete recovery from your food dependency or you wouldn't have read this far. There is hope. There is help.

ANGER

Most people I know who struggle with addiction have an underlying level of anger, even though they express it in various ways. Food-dependent individuals say,

- "Why did this happen to me?"
- "Why can't I eat like a normal person?"
- "I sit in a restaurant and see other people eating, often leaving large amounts of food. Or they eat everything and are thin."
- "What's wrong with me that I race out of control as soon as I have food in front of me?"

The only answer I can offer is that you were created different. Your enzyme system, your neurochemical system, and the way you respond are unlike those of any other person. You get angry because you are who you are. You also have choices. You can stay with your anger, think about how terrible the world is, and grumble about how badly you have been treated. Or you can learn to accept yourself as you are.

You were born different from anyone else—let that be a reason to start feeling good about yourself. You have unique skin color, shoe size, fingerprints, and hundreds of other individual features. Staying angry at your uniqueness is selling yourself short. (Later on, I'll show you how important it is to focus on your uniqueness.)

Your anger also says, "I'm mad because I can't eat a lot." This negativity is part of the addictive process. If you feel a tremendous need to want to get better so you can overeat again and lose control, you're saying you have a need to alter your mind and your perception. That's probably true now, but there is a better way.

Perhaps your anger is other directed. You're angry with your parents, the system, or the people you work with. You believe they have treated you wrong. They have created stress in your life. Maybe you have been badly and unfairly treated. Maybe your anger is justifiable. You have to move on. You have to go beyond that. Staying in your anger and feeding it with your negative thoughts intensify its power over you. You need to step toward forgiveness.

RESENTMENT

You begrudge the fact that people are pushing you into one form of action or one way of doing things. Your spouse, your friends and coworkers, or other students take advantage of you.

Because you can't speak out, you allow this resentment to stay inside and build. It's common for all of us to resent whoever puts pressure on us to change, even when we put the pressure on ourselves.

If you follow what I teach you, you can overcome your resentment. You've got to do it for yourself. The sooner you can get over your resentment, the better off you are.

BLAMING

At one time or another you've been in the blaming mode, even if you're not there now. Here's how it works. Something goes wrong, and someone has to be guilty for the error. You blame your boss. Your spouse. Your kids. The neighbors. The president or Congress or the Supreme Court.

Blaming takes the responsibility off your shoulders. You are the innocent one. By blaming, you don't have to do any soul searching or struggling with emotional problems about why you failed. Since you did nothing wrong, you don't have to give it any more concern—other than to make sure you don't get blamed by somebody else. But if you're a good blamer, you're also good at defending yourself against others' pointing fingers.

You may be highly responsible in several areas of your life, but you have a few places where you feel insecure. Those are the areas where you'll be open to blaming.

To move on, you have to think spiritually. You have to see yourself as you are before you can change.

------------------ ♥ ♥ ♥ ------------------

A vital fact about myself: I am responsible
for all my responses.

------------------ ♥ ♥ ♥ ------------------

When you can say this affirmation and mean it, you are moving out of the blaming mode. You acknowledge your responsibility to yourself and to your situation. Now you can make changes.

Share your struggle with blaming with your support person. Ask, "Am I a blamer? Do I push the responsibility for my problems on to somebody else?"

EMOTIONAL WITHDRAWAL

When people don't respond the way you want, or they hurt you or neglect you, one way to cope is to say, "I'm not going to associate with anyone. I'm going to pull back and just do my own thing." You're withdrawing not only from those who hurt you but also from everyone else.

That urge to withdraw can occur because you

- fear failure.
- fear getting caught.
- fear being different.
- fear inadequacy.
- fear not being wanted or cared about.
- fear being rejected.

Emotional withdrawal is usually an offensive move. That is, you might have withdrawn emotionally because you feared you would be rejected or be told you were not wanted. It's as if you said, "Before you run away from me, I'll run away from you." Yet as you gain more confidence in yourself and in your ability to cope, you'll stop withdrawing. You may never be the socialite of the year, but you'll be able to give of yourself to others.

DISTORTED THINKING

How do you talk to somebody who is not thinking clearly? When your chemicals are altered because of your misuse of food (and they are!), you don't perceive things the way they are in reality. You block reality from your thinking—the part of reality that prevents your seeing yourself clearly.

Before you condemn yourself for this, think about it a bit more. Somewhere in your life, distorted thinking was a way to protect yourself from hurt and pain. You used it to survive in an unhappy world. Distorted thinking served you well. But now you are in a different place in your life. You don't have to hide your inner self.

Your distorted thinking is the result of chemical changes in your brain. In your case, it probably came through your misuse of food. Such distortion also comes from stress or drugs. When you start to lose that distortion and see what's really going on, you may find it difficult to solve your problems for a while.

I urge you to work on your food-recovery program, no matter

how confused you may feel. Stay with it now. In a few months, you may need to reread this book. You'll be able to perceive the information differently by then.

As your distorted thinking and your other emotional issues diminish, you'll understand reality more clearly, and you'll become more confident and better able to cope with the other issues in your life.

27

—— ♥ ——

Underlying Thoughts

Victoria recalls that she didn't start having trouble with her weight until she was twelve or thirteen years old. Although she had never made a connection before, she said that was about the time her parents started to yell at each other. Sometimes they threw things or hit each other. Then they divorced, and she saw her father only half a dozen times in the next ten years.

As Victoria worked on her issues with food, she recalled being afraid that neither parent wanted her and that she would be put in an orphanage. "I suppose I began to overeat then," she said, "as a way of getting rid of my feelings of pain and loneliness."

I agreed that was probably true. "But, Victoria," I said, "I think you have to go back even beyond that. Before your parents started to argue a lot...think about that time. About yourself. How did you feel about who you were?"

After a lengthy silence, Victoria said, "I was shy at school, and I never thought I was as good as any of my friends." She went on to talk about her lack of self-worth.

As I listened, I believed Victoria was getting to the core of her problems. Her problems did not start with an overuse of food; they did not start with her feelings of loneliness and fear. Victoria's problems began years earlier with her low self-esteem.

Let's look at the situation in reverse order. From as far back as she could remember, Victoria thought of herself as being plain, stupid, and awkward. She had heard such words from her parents. Those were the thoughts of low self-esteem.

When Victoria was twelve, her parents began their open fights, although she admitted the tension had been there between them as long as she could remember. When they fought, her thoughts shifted into emotions, especially feelings of fear, insecurity, and abandonment. She turned to food for relief.

Victoria's story may not be typical, but the pattern is. It is the cycle of addictive, compulsive behavior. She could have used drugs (instead of food), or she could have taken on characteristics of perfectionism or become a workaholic. No matter what substance she used, Victoria was trying to soothe the feelings of pain.

In the previous chapter you read about emotions. These emotions don't just happen to you. They are the result of underlying thoughts. Because you think a particular way, you feel a particular way. Emotions follow thoughts.

For example, thoughts of low self-esteem led to feelings of inadequacy, disappointment, fear, guilt, sadness, shame, and embarrassment. Such feelings with their underlying thoughts were at work in you long before you began to misuse food. Your food dependency actually worsened them.

Food—and you might have used other drugs such as tobacco and alcohol—only worsened your situation by covering it up. The idea of being afraid—a word I use for lack of self-confidence—was present before the problem with food began. It's still there, no matter how thin you get or how you start to treat food. You have only treated your symptom (food dependency), and you have not gotten to the core issue.

The core or underlying issue for any food dependency, chemical dependency, psychological need, or addictive problem is low self-esteem.

You can reverse that process. You can build up your self-confidence—the opposite of low self-esteem. This self-confidence isn't just being good at particular tasks. It is the ability to feel good about who you *are,* whether you accomplish anything or not. I've met many excellent workers, people of outstanding ability and performance, but despite their accomplishments, they have feelings of not being good enough.

To help you build up your self-confidence, I want you to go

through two exercises. They will help you see where your self-esteem is weak.

EXERCISE 13:
HOW I SEE MYSELF

Go through the exercise, and respond with a yes or no to the descriptions. You may see yourself in several ways.

1. I am an employer or employee. My job/work/position best defines who I am. My job is a major priority. The rest of my life revolves around my work.   Yes ☐   No ☐

2. I am a parent. Having children does not mean that I actually consider them my top priority. But defining myself as a parent means that I devote an overabundance of my time, energy, and emotions to my kids and my role as a parent.   Yes ☐   No ☐

3. I am a child. I may be twenty-one or seventy. One of my roles is that of taking care of my parents or interacting with them. Even if they are dead, they influence how I live and think.
Sometimes when I speak, I can hear my mother's (or my father's) voice inside my head. I repeat things to my children that I heard from one or both parents.   Yes ☐   No ☐

4. I am a spouse. My primary role is that of a spouse. I usually think of myself as my spouse's husband or wife.   Yes ☐   No ☐

5. I am a friend. I spend much of my time with one or two special friends, whether it's dealing with their specific problems or just talking with them. I spend the majority of my energy (and often my time) in these special friendships. If I had to pick one identity role, I see myself as a loyal and caring friend.   Yes ☐   No ☐

6. I am religious. My church attendance is important, along with activities that my membership generates.   Yes ☐   No ☐

7. I am health oriented. I love exercising and learning about nutrition. I am aware of all the new information about health and fitness.   Yes ☐   No ☐

8. I am an emotionally oriented person. I am caring, and people know it. I feel deeply and sometimes wear my heart on my sleeve.   Yes ☐   No ☐

9. I am an intellectually oriented person. People who know me think of me as bright, perceptive, intellectual, and analytical. They don't call me a caring person. Occasionally, I have been called unfeeling.   Yes ☐   No ☐

10. I am a creative person. I generate ideas and new ways of doing things. I sew, paint, build things, or have a hobby that pushes me to try new things.   Yes ☐   No ☐

11. I am a sexual person. Being sexy or feeling romantic is fine with me. I'm comfortable with being (male, female) and don't compare myself to others of my gender.   Yes ☐   No ☐

12. I am a negative person. Sometimes others call me a pessimist. I don't intend to, but I tend to see the downside of most things. I see a lot of negativity in the world.   Yes ☐   No ☐

13. I am a positive person. They call me optimistic and sometimes think I'm a little naive. I tend to think that most people are good and want to help others.   Yes ☐   No ☐

14. I often feel lonely and rejected. Even when I'm with a group, I often feel alone. People say unkind, hurtful things to me. Nobody really understands me.   Yes ☐   No ☐

15. I am a person under stress. Daily, I feel tension emotionally. I also feel tension in parts of my body. I have a difficult time dealing with change, and I don't like pressure.   Yes ☐   No ☐

16. I am _____. Are there other ways you can describe yourself?   Yes ☐   No ☐

FOLLOW-UP TO EXERCISE 13

1. Discuss the results of Exercise 13 with your support person. Ask, "How do you see me?" You are not asking the person to approve or compliment you or put you down. Ask the person to check yes or no on each item.

You are trying to learn how you see yourself—not how you think you're supposed to see yourself. Your innermost thoughts about who you are affect your thought processes.

2. Look at the "yes" responses that both of you checked. Focus on these questions:

   • Is this really me?
   • Do I perceive myself correctly?
   • Is this the way I *want* to see myself?

3. Look at the "no" responses that both of you checked. Ask your support person to respond to you as you say, "This is not me because..."

4. Discuss the items about which you and your support person disagreed. Go back and ask the questions of number two.

5. Once you and your support person have decided on the characteristics that represent you, go through each answer, whether it is yes or no, and ask yourself, Who told me that was important?

For instance, suppose you decided that being an employer or employee was the most important thing. For a few minutes, relax, close your eyes, and travel back to your childhood:

   • Where did you hear that message?
   • Was it a message you heard often?
   • Which parent stressed its importance?

Think back and say, "I want to look at my friends...my pastor...my teachers...my school...my spouse...my children. Inside my mind, I want to ask them, 'Why did you say that was important?'"

Did it come from your parents, who were hard workers? Did they say that you had to make some money so you could be somebody someday and have a good job and be responsible and respected?

Who told you that being a parent was the most important? Or being a child who always responds to parents' needs? Who told you that deciding from your emotions was better? Or from your head? Perhaps one parent didn't show a lot of emotion so you learned from unspoken words that using the intellect is a better way of approaching things.

6. Discuss your answers with your support person. How did the voices speak to you then? How do they speak to you today?

7. Select your five most important answers.

Exercise 13 is to help you become more aware of how you view yourself. If you can figure out how your brain has been programmed, you can then move toward reprogramming it. How do you do that? I'll show you in the next chapter.

Vital facts about myself: I see myself with more and more clarity. I accept without criticism what I see of myself.

28

♥

Seeing Myself

You're going to use the same issues in Exercise 14 that you used in Exercise 13. This time, however, when you read the list, think about the person you want to be. That is, you would feel good about yourself if you became such a person.

If you checked that you do not see yourself as a creative person or a positive person but that is what you want to be, this time you can check yes. If you don't like something that is true of how you see yourself and you want to change that quality, this time check no.

EXERCISE 14:
HOW I WILL BE

1. I am an employer or employee.   Yes ☐   No ☐

2. I am a parent.   Yes ☐   No ☐

3. I am a child.   Yes ☐   No ☐

4. I am a spouse.   Yes ☐   No ☐

5. I am a friend.   Yes ☐   No ☐

6. I am religious.   Yes ☐   No ☐

7. I am health oriented.   Yes ☐   No ☐

8. I am an emotionally oriented person.   Yes ☐   No ☐

245

9. I am an intellectually oriented
   person.   Yes ☐   No ☐

10. I am a creative person.   Yes ☐   No ☐

11. I am a sexual person.   Yes ☐   No ☐

12. I am a negative person.   Yes ☐   No ☐

13. I am a positive person.   Yes ☐   No ☐

14. I often feel lonely and rejected.   Yes ☐   No ☐

15. I am a person under stress.   Yes ☐   No ☐

16. I am _____.   Yes ☐   No ☐

♥   ♥   ♥

From Exercise 14, select the *two* most important issues. You
will concentrate on them because they describe what you want
to be.

Affirm these two facts about yourself. First, get them into
your thoughts. Concentrate on them.

——————————   ♥   ♥   ♥   ——————————

Vital facts about myself: I am _____.

I am _____.

——————————   ♥   ♥   ♥   ——————————

Second, I want to remind you how your brain stores information. If you have been told, "You are lazy," and you accept it
as a true statement, it won't matter whether that's actually a
true fact or not. It won't matter how hard you work at trying to
prove you're not lazy. You have already stored the information
that says, "I am a lazy person."

Please don't try to deny these "truths" you've accepted because that doesn't work. No matter how much praise or recognition you receive, your brain has not changed. In your
thinking, you are a lazy person. So how did you cope with the
painfulness of the laziness? You turned to food or some other
substance.

Now you are ready to change. Here's how it works.

Tell yourself, "I am industrious. I work hard." Repeat affirmations about yourself. Say them to yourself again and again until they are imprinted or stored in your brain *and* they have replaced the earlier, negative messages.

As you work and produce, you receive praise and recognition. Eventually, if you get more messages that say, "I am a hard worker," instead of, "I am lazy," your memory storage shifts. You slowly accept this new information.

EXERCISE 15:
TWO GOALS

Decide on the two most important goals from Exercise 14 you need to address to prevent your emotions from triggering your need to eat. For example, you may decide you need to strengthen your relationship with your spouse by discussing issues you have learned in this book and to become a more positive person.

G O A L

1: _____

_____

G O A L

2: _____

_____

EXERCISE 16:
HOW I CAN MAKE CHANGES

The following material provides action steps for meeting each of your two most important goals.

1. I spend more time with _____. If your goal is to be a parent, obviously you'd better write in your kids.

2. I spend more time to _____.
Maybe it's time to go for a walk, to share, or to be quiet. For example, if you are stressed but your goal is to be a parent,

maybe you need to spend more time to enjoy a hobby before you spend time with the kids.

3. I spend less time _____.
Obviously, if you need more time for what you identified in numbers one and two, you're going to spend less time at something else. You have only a certain amount of time. Are you going to spend less time being with friends or watching TV?

4. I treat *(name)* _____ as a more supportive person. (Do not name your support person.) Perhaps you feel that your spouse nags you all the time. Or maybe you're a child, and your parents demand too much from you. Or maybe one of your close friends berates you and criticizes you often. Decide to give the person support. Listen to the person's needs, confusion, and pain. When he starts criticizing you, ask yourself, Why does he criticize? Why does he care enough to complain about these things?

You can begin to see that the person isn't against you. She cares. She wants the best for you and wants you to be the best you can be.

At this point, you're not seeking more effective communication. You're not attempting to fix anything. Concentrate on this thought: He complains because he cares. You must matter, or he wouldn't get all riled up.

What if you turned around and treated her supportively? If you affirmed her? If you showed her that you were with her in her struggles?

The next time a significant person in life starts complaining, here's what I urge you to do. First, listen so that you hear the complaint. Then say, "Okay, I understand. I'll do whatever I can to be different." You have been supportive by hearing the complaint and responding positively.

5. I share more time _____. You're going to open up and tell more of your failures, fears, inadequacies, and wants. You may do this with your support person or the one you've chosen to support more. Rearrange your life so that you can share more time.

6. I listen more to _____. Communication includes listening and sharing, which means listening so that you actually hear and absorb what the person is

saying. You may think that the talk is about superficial things, and that may frustrate you. Listen anyway.

You now have taken definite steps that lead you toward becoming different—becoming the person you want to be. You need to be different to affect the way you think about yourself. If you begin to change the way you see yourself and think about yourself and you change the actions and you get validation from others, you will change.

29

— ♥ —

Moving in Stages

Recovery from food-related problems is a process. If you are willing to work until you are fully recovered, you will go through four distinct stages.

If you know what to expect ahead of time, you can be better prepared and learn the pitfalls and danger points. Your support person, spouse, parents, and children can also benefit from knowing about these stages in your recovery and growth.

STAGE 1:
"I'M NOT DOING IT..."

At this stage you concentrate on eliminating your compulsive behavior. You think and talk about what you don't do any longer. Generally, this process takes up to six months after you've discontinued your misuse of food and eliminated any other addictive forms of behavior.

Here are characteristics common to persons in Stage 1.

1. You still think about food even though you no longer overeat

Pleasant memories return:

- "Ahh, I used to eat a pound of chocolate a week."
- "I'll never forget the tantalizing smell of Joe's

French fries and special hamburgers. I always had
to eat several helpings."
- "Nothing tastes quite like four dozen fried shrimp."
- "Those flaky pie crusts. They melted in my mouth."

You'll think of special meals and the good times associated
with overeating (and tend not to think of the results and the
bad times). At this point, you need to remain aware of the
battles you face. Old habits can strike at you through your
feelings, yearnings, desires, and mood shifts.

2. You have food cravings

The word *cravings* may confuse you. Craving means that
you would, in certain situations, think about and yearn for all
kinds of food. You have daydreams of a wonderful fattening
meal of sweets. Maybe you wake up in the middle of the night
with dreams of the best Christmas meal you've ever had.

If you have these cravings, it is all right. It does happen to
some individuals. The neurochemicals affected by your food
misuse are now rearranging themselves. They're bouncing
around a bit. One day, you feel perfectly fine, and the next day,
you wonder how you hit bottom.

Cravings are common during the initial weight-loss period.
Generally, they occur between sixty and ninety days into the
weight-loss program. Your brain is readapting, the chemicals
in the brain are changing, and feedback is beginning to be
altered.

You need to supplement your weight loss with your eating
plan. You are now going on a lifetime "diet for the brain." You
need to make sure that the neurotransmitters that have become depleted with weight loss and cause cravings are altered.
Keep your caloric total the same, but switch food types as
described in your self-selected eating program.

3. You feel lonely and confused

It takes time, but your brain chemistry will change. In the
meantime, no matter how committed you are to recovery, a
part of you still doesn't want to stop overeating. There will be
times in your recovery when you'll feel as if you are all alone.

And when you are lonely or confused, you find dozens of reasons to binge "just this once."

4. You feel tempted to overeat again

Watch for the little temptations that can sidetrack you. You'll find reasons to overeat every day: if the phone keeps ringing and you can't get any work done; if the phone doesn't ring and you get distracted waiting for someone to call; if the weather gets too warm or too cold; or if the dogs in the neighborhood bark and keep you awake.

5. You have trouble getting in touch with your true feelings

Because you haven't been in touch with your real self for a long time, you may not know what is a real emotion and what isn't. Do I really feel this way? you may ask. Real emotions are the feelings you would experience if your brain were now a balanced brain. The imbalanced brain causes feelings that seem absolutely "real," but they are a result of the misperception of reality.

6. You often feel frustrated

Quite likely you'll struggle with your emotions and say,

- "Sometimes I feel like giving up."
- "When does this end?"
- "Nobody cares anyway, so why don't I just hang it up?"
- "At first, I felt so confident. Now I wonder why I wanted to change anyway."
- "I just don't feel like going on."

7. You tend to feel that nobody is giving you positive responses for your efforts

You feel as if friends and family don't understand what's going on inside your mind. The truth is, they probably don't understand. And because they don't, they don't realize how difficult it is for you to deal with some issues in your life.

From the people who are important to you, you get no rewards (praise) unless they realize that you need the encouragement. Unless you tell them what you need, here is your situation: You've given up a reward (overeating, which medicated your bad feelings), and nobody recognizes what you're going through. You feel terrible when you expected to feel wonderful. However, if you start doing things positively, you'll get praise for your positive actions.

When I've spoken with families of persons in recovery, they've said things such as:

- "Well, we were afraid that it wouldn't last."
- "She has tried before, you know, a hundred times, and if we make too big a deal of it and she fails again..."
- "I thought he knew I was proud of him. I told him so when he started the program. I didn't realize he needed all that ongoing encouragement."

Here are my suggestions for you to bear in mind as you work through Stage 1. Stick close to your activity plan, eating plan, and support system. You are dealing with neurochemical issues. This stage will probably last from two to eight weeks—and you may feel this strongly. It will then tend to decrease, perhaps even go away for weeks. You may have a less-intense recurrence near the end of your first six-month period.

Start doing positive things. Focus on the positive changes you're making instead of looking at what you are no longer doing. Instead of saying, "I'm doing really good because I'm not overeating," say,

- "I'm doing good because I'm spending more time with the family."
- "I'm thinking clearer."
- "I like life more than ever."

Work on your positive affirmations.

--------------------------------   ♥ ♥ ♥   --------------------------------

A vital fact about myself: I stay with my
recovery plan, no matter how my emotions
fluctuate.

--------------------------------   ♥ ♥ ♥   --------------------------------

STAGE 2: "I FEEL..."

One person referred to Stage 2 as the killer stage. In Stage 1 many people rely on self-will or willpower to make it through. They're tough and aggressive people. They focus on not overeating, but they do make it through. Stage 2 requires reliance on self-discipline instead of self-will.

"As long as you focus on what you're *not* doing," I've told thousands of people, "you're going to get in trouble."

Stage 2 usually occurs around six months, and it can last up to two years if you don't follow the program you have been setting up in these chapters. If you follow the program, the severity of your problems decreases almost daily.

You start experiencing neurohormonal effects. Your brain releases hormones and changes chemicals, and it often feels confused about the "normal" level of neurochemicals. This inrush or retention of chemicals causes your emotions to change without reason. One day, you feel lighthearted. The next day, you're severely depressed, but you can't identify anything that depressed you.

Supportive friends, who don't understand what is going on, exhort, "Just get hold of yourself. Hang in there." They speak as if it's a simple matter of making up your mind about what to do. They don't realize that you feel depressed because your brain is trying to balance itself.

Here are the common characteristics of Stage 2.

1. You have frequent mood changes

You may be doing fine, but all of a sudden you wake up one day and say, "I want a couple of chocolate doughnuts. I'm depressed."

Mood changes come about because of several components in addiction. One is the neurochemical changes. Chemical changes in the brain affect the hormonal system. Contrary to what some may think, the hormonal system isn't significant only for females. But hormonal change is both common and significant in males and in adolescents.

It works this way. If you are supplying chemicals from your food or from other substances, your remarkably efficient brain says, "I don't need to do all of this work. I'm getting the chemicals from the outside." And it slows down production of neurochemicals. When you stop providing these neurochemicals from food, your body is slow in catching up and cries out, "Help! We need more."

That's a scary position to be in, and it will probably happen to you. Your best weapon of defense is to be aware and to get yourself ready. You can be alert to the warning signs, and you can also take action.

2. You forget that *you* are the problem

This is a problem not in self-will but in self-discipline.

self-will (or **willpower**): attempting to discontinue an addictive behavior on your own, telling yourself you can do it without help

self-discipline: carrying out the actions that bring about change, the willingness to act once you have committed yourself to a program

The going-it-alone attitude doesn't usually work because your food dependency is physiologically and psychologically stronger. And as I've pointed out, your overeating has been an automatic reaction to various triggers.

Self-discipline is crucial. Your neurochemicals became imbalanced through consistent, long-term behavior. The reverse, which is neurochemical health, also comes through consistent, long-term behavior.

3. Fear is one of your strongest emotions

Fear lurks everywhere in your life:

- "I don't think that our relationship is going to make it."

- "I don't feel I can ever be a good mother (father)."
- "How will I ever be able to get along with my parents?"
- "I'm going to lose my job. I know I am."
- "Nobody wants to be my friend. I'm going to be alone and deserted."
- "What if I can't hold out? What if I go back to overeating again?"

4. You may become a little paranoid

Your confidence drops, and you're convinced that everyone has rejected you or soon will. The rejection creates a lot of anger.

5. Self-pity fills in the vacant holes

You moan, "Nobody cares. I've done all this hard work, and people just pick on me or draw back. They don't treat me any nicer or act as if they know I'm changed. I feel so angry, and I don't know what to do about it."

6. Your denial system kicks in

You might be tempted to overeat and say,

- "I'm not really going to go back to overeating again."
- "Just this once. It's a special occasion."
- "You know, to give myself a little courage in facing all those people."

7. You may become a blamer

You get upset and blame the weather, the federal government, friends, bosses, financial status, or daily pressures. You can come up with hundreds of reasons why your recovery program won't work.

You may even self-blame: "I'm a failure. That's all I've ever been. I've never succeeded on any diet. What makes me think I can succeed now?"

Part of your emotional swings has to do with your basic

personality, but the chemicals in your brain certainly exacerbate them. Recommit yourself to your eating plan, your activity program, and your support system. Work on spiritual and self-esteem issues.

These are all issues that, combined with the triggers, you'll find of great importance. Keep saying to yourself, "I know this is happening. I reexamine my triggers. I redefine my issues."

8. Your thought towers involve a lifelong process

If you stay with it, the day will come—not too far in the future—when you will automatically have control over your thought towers. For now, I urge you to do your exercises faithfully. Later, you won't have to go through every one of the steps as you do now.

You'll be able to say to yourself, "This thought triggers this particular behavior." It becomes an almost subconscious action as you continue to make changes.

--------- ♥ ♥ ♥ ---------

A vital fact about myself: Despite my fears,
I stay with my recovery program.

--------- ♥ ♥ ♥ ---------

STAGE 3: "I HIT THE WALL..."

In the beginning of Stage 3, you can feel constantly depressed, scared, fearful, or anxious, or you can have mood changes. You can expect these changes sometime between seven and ten months after you stop overeating.

You may develop a negative attitude. You may develop a serious problem with seeing things the way other people do. If these things happen, the consequences can be the loss of your job, the breakup of your marriage or relationship, and/or the destruction of friendships.

You may say, "I've been eating properly for nearly a year. I'm depressed. I know I don't feel particularly good about myself or my life."

Stage 3 is the bottom of the pits. You tend not to feel good about anything and wonder if all your work has been worth it.

You may return to your overeating. A number of people go six months to a year or two years without overeating. Then it hits. This period can be dangerous.

Perhaps the best way to describe how most people going through diet recovery respond is to tell you about Tim, who was an overeater.

"I was overweight for twenty-one years," Tim said when he came to me the first time. Eight months later he reached his desired weight through a program at the Diet Center. He came to see me a few months later. On one visit he looked thoroughly rejected and downhearted.

"What's wrong?" I asked.

"I failed. I blew it."

"What do you mean?"

Shame was written all over his face. He couldn't look me in the eyes. "I binged on a bag of cookies. A large bag."

I waited, but that was all he said. "Tim, I understand that much. But you said you failed. Tell me about it."

Shock and then confusion appeared on his face. "Didn't you hear me? *I binged on cookies.*"

"You know, Tim," I said, "you told me a few months ago that you had a terrible relationship with your wife, and she was ready to walk out on you. You said that your two sons screamed that they hated you. You were barely holding on to your job. You didn't have a relationship with God. You told me that you never felt confident about anything and didn't like yourself very much. You said that eating helped you forget how bad you felt. Is all of that true?"

He nodded.

"Then I don't understand," I said. "Over the course of your visits, you've been telling me that you have made all these changes. Why, a month ago you told me that you felt really close to your wife and two boys. And now you're saying that you're a failure? Is that true? Are you a failure? Really a failure?"

"Well, I . . . I feel like a failure," he mumbled.

"Tim, you ate compulsively for over twenty years before you

stopped. Now you relapse by bingeing on a bag of cookies, and you decide you want to give up—"

"I don't want to give up. I *have* given up—"

"Really? To me, this isn't a story about failure. You've given me a success story."

Tim opened his mouth to respond and then shook his head slowly. "I . . . I . . . I never . . . never thought . . . I mean, all I could see was failure."

To this day, nine years later, Tim hasn't gone back to bingeing. He had a period that some refer to as "hitting the wall." He relapsed slightly, and he struggled with guilt and failure and various other negative emotions. Fortunately, he was able to hear what I said, and then he moved on in his recovery to the fourth and final stage.

Marsha was a compulsive dieter for at least ten years. She finally underwent a stomach bypass operation and lost well over 150 pounds. However, the surgery was only partially successful, and she has a lifetime of minor health problems. She has not regained her former weight, but she has not gotten into any exercise program or done any of the things I recommend in this book.

Marsha discontinued her food abuse, but she did nothing else. Not long ago, she told me, "Joel, it's been ten years this month since I lost all that weight."

I congratulated her, of course.

She attends three twelve-step meetings a week and can tell you anything you want to know about calories, fat content, and cholesterol.

Yet as I walked away I thought, *Marsha is an excellent candidate for the most miserable person I have ever known.* In the past decade, she has gone through two divorces. Her three kids won't talk to her. Worse than that, she is a controlling, bitter, angry person.

Is Marsha successful because she hasn't abused food for ten years? If that was her only goal, I'd say yes. But to look at her as a woman who wants to be loved and needed, who wants to live a joyful life, I'd have to say that she failed. She concentrates on what she's *not* doing—not overeating—but apparently, she has done little toward finding happiness in life.

By contrast, Tim is far more successful, even though he

relapsed once. Even if he relapsed five times (and I'm not condoning that!), he learned from his failures. Tim hit Stage 3 and didn't get trapped there. Marsha is trapped in Stage 1 —she's never moved on.

In Stage 3, what causes individuals to hit the wall?

1. You may have a genetic problem

You have chemical imbalances acquired from your parents. They prevent you from feeling good. Genetic recovery is hard, but it's not impossible.

You may require medication to control your neurochemical alterations. But don't grab on to that solution too quickly. Try the plan you set up for yourself in this book. If you still face mood swings or bouts with depression, see your physician right away. (I encourage you to get two opinions; even an expert can sometimes miss something crucial.)

2. You may come from a dysfunctional family

Generational problems may affect you. Frequently, abuse issues have surfaced.

3. You may have transferred your addictions

Most people in recovery programs are in Stage 3 today. Your neurochemicals haven't changed because you didn't follow neurochemical recovery techniques.

You may have stopped overeating, but now you are a workaholic or a chain smoker. You transfer the unmet needs so you can satisfy them with another form of addiction. *You never deal with basic problems*.

Earlier, we discussed dysfunctional family problems and transfer of addictions; you can deal with the issues as I've described in the book. If you follow the activities, eating plans, and behavioral suggestions, hitting the wall should not be a long-term problem for you.

♥ ♥ ♥

A vital fact about myself: I focus on my successes and not my failures.

♥ ♥ ♥

STAGE 4: "I'M FREE..."

Stage 4 completes the cycle. As a fully recovered person, you will still have problems, but you have learned techniques for gaining control over your life. You now make your own choices.

You are free.

30

— ♥ —

Relapse—Part of Recovery?

Relapse is an intimidating word. Unfortunately, it happens.
Does this describe you? For weeks you've been making progress. Then unexpectedly, something happens and you binge.
"What is going on with me?" you wail. "I was doing so well."
First, before you are too hard on yourself, recognize that
relapse is a common occurrence in recovery from the diseases
of dependency. Food dependency is a form of chemical dependency.
I don't like relapse anymore than the person who relapses
does. It can be devastating, and it's hard to get your support
people back unless they understand. If relapse happens to you,
please remember this: Relapse is one misstep in a long journey. I've seen it happen to a large number of people who make
successful recoveries.
Second, relapse and its repercussions will be less troublesome if you focus on who you are. Isn't relapse simply going
back to your former life-style? You have to come a long way
before you can go back. You have made progress!
Third, if you relapse, take a careful look at the areas you
have worked on in this book. Honestly ask yourself these
questions:

- Have I faithfully followed my exercise program?
- Have I faithfully followed my activity program?
- Have I faithfully followed my eating plan?
- Have I faithfully worked on my thought towers?

• Have I faithfully gone to meetings?
• Have I faithfully met with my support person?

(*Faithfully* doesn't mean perfectly; it does mean that you have tried and done these things with commitment and regularity.)

Fourth, you'll help yourself if you ask, What happened in my life? What brought this on? Don't focus on your guilt, your lack of willpower, or your shortcomings. Don't tell yourself you are weak, powerless, and useless. Go back to your thought towers. Get in touch with the thoughts that created negative emotions of anger, denial, and hopelessness.

Fifth, use your support system. Talk to them. Let them help you. Tell them the conclusions you have reached: "I relapsed because..."

Sixth, listen to their feedback. Then backtrack. Backtrack happens when you see the steps that led to your relapse.

Seventh, don't continue in your relapse while you say, "It's going to get better. I'm only going to try it for a while, and then I'll get back on track again."

These words are often spoken in Stage 2 when persons in recovery have a certain amount of confidence. They think they can go back and face huge amounts of food and not give in. When they give in, they deny the power of their old habits and say, "One time...just today..."

If you are tempted to overeat once, remember that overeating has been your major problem area for a long time. Do you honestly want to get back into that abusive cycle again? Can you honestly think of one good reason for going back? There are none.

SIX RED FLAGS OF RELAPSE

In your recovery, you will encounter the Red Flags of Relapse. I want to warn you about them. They take place before you relapse. Watch for them. Share these Red Flags with your support person and perhaps with your spouse or family members.

1. Unclear thinking

You're making progress, and then suddenly, you're confused. Your clear path isn't so obvious any longer. You wonder,

- Where do I go now?
- How can I handle this?
- What *are* my goals?
- What is happening to me?
- Is this what I really want?

Life has become fuzzy, and you're not putting things together anymore. Your support people can sometimes see what is happening and may even tell you. But if you're thinking unclearly, you may not be able to hear them unless you're prepared for this Red Flag.

2. Sleep disturbances

This Red Flag shows itself in numerous ways:

- You're sleeping more or not enough.
- You're tired, but you can't fall asleep.
- You're having trouble staying asleep, or you lie awake until morning.
- You have to force yourself to get out of bed in the morning.

3. Uncontrolled emotions

You're normally even tempered, but you find yourself getting angry—a lot. You're frustrated. You battle

- depression or anxiety.
- sadness.
- shame.
- insecurities.

These emotional issues intrude, and you say, "I don't know what's going on."

4. Physical symptoms

You develop backaches and headaches. Lately you've been feeling extremely tired. You're not really sick, but you just don't feel good. You have pains in various places. If you're a chronic pain patient, your hurting increases.

5. Spiritual distancing

One day you think, *I used to feel so good about God and my faith. Now I wonder if my spiritual dimension is important anymore.* You get angry with God. You realize that you're distancing yourself from God and from God's people.

6. Stress sensitivity

You used to handle enormous amounts of stress, but you've become highly sensitive. It doesn't take much before you are stressed.

♥ ♥ ♥

Those are the Six Red Flags of Relapse. If you see any one of them begin to develop, go into action. Here are things you can do for yourself:

- Get support.
- Talk to somebody, especially your support people.
- Check your thoughts; work on your thought tower.
- Check up on your spirituality—how you view life and what you expect.
- Review the material in this book, which includes following the programs you have set up.
- Practice the affirmation of your vital facts by reading and repeating them.

FREQUENT RELAPSE

You've handled your eating well, but then you relapse. If you don't straighten out and get back on track and stay on track, you're in trouble. If you relapse every few weeks or after two months, you're in big trouble. I don't want to frighten you, but I do want to warn you.

Frequent relapse means your food dependency is becoming more progressive. This is true even if you say, "I'm eating less," or "I only overeat once in a while." It is becoming progressive because inside you're losing hope. You're developing a system of denial.

Frequent relapse means you've got to get more aggressive. Take more action steps. You may need a lot of help from every part of your support system. Ask for help. Don't be ashamed because of the relapses, but use them as determination to reach out for help.

Frequent relapse means you want to quit. DON'T QUIT! You are probably closer to victory than you think. Give it one more big boost. Remember how miserable you were before. Even if you feel you are more miserable now, you aren't. It just feels that way because your neurochemicals are bouncing around.

♥ ♥ ♥

Vital facts about myself: I guard against relapse. *But* if I relapse, I forgive myself and go on.

♥ ♥ ♥

31

♥

Coping with the Real World

I'm a husband. I have three children, all girls. I know the hassles of child rearing, of priorities, of finances, and of all the usual issues that come about from living in the real world.

Your real world is different from mine. I may not understand all your specific issues—and no one does except you—but I'd like you to look at some issues that I predict you'll encounter. I'd like to offer you insight into ways to handle them so that the day-to-day issues won't become major stumbling blocks to trip you up and pitch you back into food dependency.

YOUR NEW LIFE

You're living a new life

If you have followed this book, you've been challenged in areas where you may not want to be challenged. You've learned more about yourself, although you're inexperienced in coping with new values and ideals. You know at least that the old way of handling the problems won't work for the new you.

You haven't eliminated stress

Life *is* stress. You have discovered new stresses—but ones that are manageable.

You will confront unmet expectations

Because you changed, you got it into your mind that others would change, too. You assumed your friends and relatives would respond differently. But they didn't, and you might be confused.

You need less-immediate rewards

In your old ways of thinking, when you felt low, you turned to food (and you might also have turned to drugs, alcohol, or some other substance or behavior). You did something—usually put something into your body—to make yourself feel less pain or give you a temporary good feeling. Now you can be less compulsive when you are down and eat more sensibly to cope with emotional issues.

Your highs and lows are different

You don't get as low as you used to, and you don't get as high when you're feeling good. If you're responding like most people, you're discovering that your emotions are more consistent. That may give you cause for concern.

David said, "I had felt so bad for so many years that when I started to feel good, I didn't know how to react. For several days I had no depression, and I hadn't been without depression for at least ten years. It took me a long time to feel good about feeling good."

You have changed. I want you to be able to celebrate that change. Here is your affirmation:

——————— ♥ ♥ ♥ ———————

Vital facts about myself: I have overcome my food dependency. I am a new person.

——————— ♥ ♥ ♥ ———————

AREAS OF DIFFICULTY

You may want to believe that once you've stepped into your new life, you'll never have problems again. You'll have problems, but you'll have healthy coping devices. You'll be aware of the pitfalls and struggles.

Remember that your real world is different from anybody

else's, which includes the way you were raised, the way you respond to crisis and happiness, and the choices you make. You can't rely totally on your support person or anyone else; you will have to apply these insights to your new life.

From my experience in working with persons recovering from food dependency, I have consistently seen some major areas of difficulty. Let's look at each one.

You will learn that people will fail you

Perhaps your original support person didn't work out. You can't understand why people aren't responding the way you want. You feel let down. There are several reasons.

1. You are now different. You perceive things more clearly. You are standing closer to reality than ever before. That doesn't solve all your problems. You may still perceive issues differently from others. For instance, you may think, *I've stayed on my weight-loss program and lost the pounds I wanted. I no longer abuse food. They should be praising me and feeling excited about what's happened.* Unfortunately, people have so many problems of their own that often they can't get in touch with those of others. They aren't tuned in when others recover.

2. You feel rejected by some of your friends. The friends that you used to socialize with aren't available anymore. You're too sensitive to problems—not just yours—and you may make many of them feel uncomfortable. They're still denying they need help, so they don't want to be around you. If they don't have a food-dependency problem, they may not know how to support you because they don't understand your disease.

3. You feel as if you get nothing but criticism. People tend to focus on your weaknesses and faults. Don't believe them. Don't accept your shortcomings as your major sense of identity.

4. You may realize people are treating you differently. Frankly, people just don't always understand others.

It all comes down to this reality: People fail other people. If you put your faith in other human beings, you won't make it. That's partially why I stress spirituality as a vital ingredient in your life. Even if people let you down, God won't fail.

Others have their own issues to cope with. And they do need to take care of themselves first. I've put this to practical use. I've learned that when people criticize me, two things are important. First, I need to find out if there is any legitimacy to the criticism. If there is, I'd better listen and make some changes. Second, I need to ask myself, Why did they need to criticize me? What are they getting out of it? Are they feeling better about themselves by putting me down? That's how certain individuals operate.

You will eventually end up in places or situations where you misused food before

You may be with friends who do not understand; they may be ignorant of your problems. You may need to choose new friends. But before you get in such situations, plan how you're going to handle them. You can have a ready-made excuse to leave. You can have support from a friend or relative.

If you use those three things—planning, a ready-made excuse, and a support person—you'll be able to handle most situations. I'm not encouraging you to go into situations where you previously binged. But you won't be able to avoid them altogether. You won't want to avoid wedding receptions, all parties, and dinners at restaurants. Withdrawing isn't healthy. Carefully consider situations where you know you're going to be tempted and prepare yourself to cope.

You will likely have some sexual frustration

One of the most significant elements of the real world in recovery is sexual frustration.

1. You may be impaired because of your abuse of food, and additional weight can adversely affect sexual performance.

2. The relationship has changed between you and your spouse. Previously, one of you felt used or angry. Or if you did have sex, it was more out of an obligation to the other than from your own desires. Now you've recovered and are ready for sexual activity again. Issues may exist that will take time to clear up. Five or six months after discontinuing food dependency, some individuals are still resolving their sexual problems—including being able to perform and getting their feelings sorted out. Be willing to give it a little time.

3. You may not find the level of support you want. In some husband-wife relationships, one person has been food dependent and now has changed. If that is you, your expectation level is probably high.

What about your spouse? Is your spouse food dependent or addicted to a negative form of behavior? Realizing you have changed, your spouse may expect to see tremendous changes in you—more than you can deliver. However, some things don't change. Your basic personality is the same. You may be learning to communicate and offer support, but even these things happen slowly.

Your emotional responses don't change that quickly. It takes time—weeks at least—for you to change your thoughts so that you can change your feelings. Consequently, your spouse may feel disappointed or angry unless you are able to share your ongoing struggle.

Just as you need to be respected, your spouse needs to feel your respect and support before the sexual experience can be positive. You show your respect by the way you communicate, share, and listen.

I urge you to find ways to express your respect and your desire for intimacy and to make efforts to be tender. Understand also that people operate on different time schedules. Some hit their stride by jumping out of bed at the crack of dawn, and others don't even feel sleepy until it's nearly dawn. If you and your spouse seem to be living in different time zones, how do you cope? Sharing and talking about it will help. Even if you're not comfortable discussing it, it's a vital part of the relationship. If you want to get rid of your frustrations, talking is one of the best ways to resolve them.

You will feel stress

These are real-world stresses.

Check your identity. Consider how you spend your time. Previously, I've referred to the social, physical, relational, educational/vocational, and spiritual elements. Where do you spend your time? If you've got them balanced, you're still in control when any area feels stressed. You can still be victorious.

Balance the amount of time and energy (thoughts, too) you devote to the various areas.

Draw a circle and divide it into five equal parts. The whole circle represents you. Each part represents 20 percent of your identity. Now indicate how much time, energy, and thought you devote to each of the five areas. If 20 percent of you is job stressed, that means 80 percent of you isn't stressed. You're balanced, and you're going to be all right.

But what if 80 percent of your time, energy, and thoughts is spent at your job, and the other 20 percent is divided among the other areas? If you're job stressed, 80 percent of you is stressed, and 20 percent of you isn't stressed. You're badly out of balance. You won't think appropriately or realistically. Being out of balance in one area affects every other area of your life. You need to get balance so that you're in control.

There are two types of stress. One stress is the type I can identify—it's objective. With some reflection, I can figure out what it is. Suppose I am in my office, and I look out the window and see that I have a flat tire on my car. I'm stressed about the flat tire because I want to get home right away, but I can't. How do I handle objective stress? Usually, I can take care of it. With the flat tire, it's simple. Either I call somebody to give me a ride home, or I change the tire. However, until I've done something to make a change, I'm going to have a problem and be subject to objective stress.

Objective stress says, "I know the problem, and I'm going to change it." When you encounter stress that you can identify, you can do something to change the situation. You can deal with it.

The other type of stress is subjective. Subjective stress says, "I don't know what I'm stressed about. I can't pinpoint it. I feel insecure...unsure...anxious. I can't define what I'm feeling." It may be stress to which you think there is no solution. Most stresses have solutions. The problem is, you don't have the solution.

If you have subjective stress, you need to examine your spiritual values. It may help you to memorize a prayer that members of AA and other twelve-step programs regularly recite. Written by Reinhold Niebuhr, it is called the Serenity Prayer: "God, give us grace to accept with serenity the things that cannot be changed, courage to change the things which should be changed, and the wisdom to distinguish the one from the other."

In learning to accept what you can't change, you may need to accept the reality that your spouse is the way he or she is. Your children are who they are. Your parents probably aren't going to become different. Your dysfunctional childhood is part of your past, and it won't ever be different. That's acceptance. The sooner you say, "That's the way things are," the sooner your stress goes away.

You may turn away from religion

Attaining spiritual health is tough for a lot of people. There are four things I'd like to talk to you about if you sincerely feel turned off by religion or spirituality.

1. You turn away from religion because it takes time to begin to understand God and to believe. Yet having faith in a power beyond yourself is essential for your recovery. Spirituality is a growth process that goes forward until the day you die. Just don't give up.

2. You turn away from religion because the supporters of a religion or denomination tell you that truth exists. If you have trouble accepting truth, are you trying to redefine it to something you can accept? With the increased interest in cults and Eastern religion, I hear more and more these days about "your truth" and "my truth" as if truth can be bent to fit anyone. A better way is to realize that some universal, objective truths exist. Are you having trouble accepting that there are some universal truths? If so, you need to do some serious self-examining. Ask yourself why you have this difficulty. You may discover that you have done this because of your personal needs. But when you concentrate on "my truth," you will discover that such a system will ultimately fail you.

3. You turn away from religion because of the style of worship. You may need to find another style of worship. Change denominations or churches. One church doesn't fit everybody. If you've been in one type of church and you're uncomfortable, you probably don't belong there. Search until you find a place that meets your needs.

4. You turn away from religion because you haven't found a "healing minister." By that I mean a pastor who doesn't condemn you or make you feel you're on a greasy slide toward hell when you're not. Talk to somebody who cares and understands people. Share with that person.

You may feel that your relationships aren't close or intimate

You're having trouble with relationship issues—whether with your parents, kids, spouse, or friends. You say, "I wanted that closeness and set it as one of my goals. All we have is a kind of peaceful coexistence." You don't scream at each other anymore, but you admit, "We don't have a close relationship, and I need that."

Why do you have problems with close relationships? Consider these possibilities.

1. You set up impossible expectations. When spouses get back together and seek a close relationship, they set up wrong goals, or they seek too much from the relationship too soon. And one person fails.

For example, you may decide on this goal: I want my spouse to be romantic, caring, and supportive and to always respect me. That's an impossible situation. If your spouse fails once or in one area, you start distancing: "You failed! You let me down!" The reality is that you tried to get too much. You need to take the crawl-walk-run approach.

Generally, for couples to reach a true level of intimacy after one of them has been involved in food dependency, it takes four to five years. It may take a lifetime.

Concentrate on making progress in the areas of intimacy and respect. You can then enjoy each other more.

2. You have been burned before, so you're cautious. You tried to get close, but it didn't work. Or perhaps you have been free from your food dependency for a period of months. Then other people decide to jump in and be supportive, and all of a sudden you relapse again. They withdraw. You have to talk to them and share to get past that one.

3. You don't tell others how or what to give you. You have to share your needs with them.

I'll give you a personal example. I tend to be more private, but my wife tends to be more public. Now, I also like to have control of my busy schedule. My wife enjoys time with people. Socially we go out together, but it's not something I would generally think of. Because Vickie has a need for more socialization, we go. However, if Vickie schedules time for us to get with another couple and tells me, she finds me a little distant. When she feels that coming from me, she backs off. Then we have a problem. How do we work it out?

Suppose Vickie said, "Joel, we need to get with the Martins. I really like being with them. When can you fit that in?" If she left the matter hanging until I replied, I probably wouldn't get back to her for about a year. We have found that it works best if Vickie says to me, "What would be the best day this week for us to get with the Martins?"

Why does this work? First, I have time to think of my schedule and see how I can spend time with the Martins and still do what I feel I need to do. Second, I have a choice. I decide on the time that suits me best. I can then prepare my workload to be ready for it.

Question: How did Vickie know to approach me that way?

Answer: I told her.

I had to tell Vickie the best way to work with me. She doesn't read my mind, and she wants to be intimate in ways that both of us can be true to our basic personalities. So I had to say things to her such as:

- "When I mess things up, wait until the next day to talk to me about it. Otherwise I may be too defensive."
- "Tell me the names of the people you'd like us to develop a close friendship with."
- "Tell me how I can best support you because I don't know."

4. You think you may be codependent—and you may be. You may be in a situation where it's difficult for you to understand healthy relationships. As a codependent, you turned to someone else to make you feel happy. Because you were unable to find happiness yourself, that labels you codependent.

Jerry was codependent. He was heartbroken when his wife left him. He had been verbally abusive, he finally admitted, and was away from home more than necessary. For weeks after she left, Jerry refused to see where he had failed. One day he said, "You know, now I realize that I've always looked to someone to provide for all my emotional needs. No wonder my wife left me. Nobody could do what I expected of her."

If that situation describes the old you, you were codependent.

5. You need to look at personality issues and communication. Go back to chapter 22 and reread about the Bear, Bunny, Banshee, Bird, and Buffalo. Rethink issues such as control and power.

Everybody communicates in a fashion based on personality. I may be a direct person who says, "Hey, can you take the trash out for me?" I feel comfortable saying that, and I don't feel I'm making a demand. Another person may say, "The trash stinks. It's been in the kitchen six days. I'd appreciate it if you'd consider that this stuff spreads germs. The kids are getting a lot of colds and sniffles." This person uses guilt or manipulation to get the other to take the trash out. Part of it may be a communication technique, but it's largely a matter of personality.

Couples, families, and friends can do so much toward improving relationships if they can learn to say, "This is the best way for me to...," or "What's the best way for me to approach you about...?"

Ask. Don't try to change anyone. Ask, "What's the best way?" You also need to say, "With my personality...," or "Because of the kind of person I am, I'm having a little trouble with that." These statements and questions open the door for better communication.

You may be persistently anxious or depressed

You're going to be up at times and down at others. But if you regularly and consistently feel anxious or depressed, you need to think about some things.

1. You have to communicate more. Convey more clear messages of how you feel and what you want and need. Instead of telling another, "You're not meeting my needs," say, "Let me explain to you the best way that you can help me meet my needs." Don't put others on the defensive if they're not doing what you want or if they're doing something you don't like. Simply saying, "Here's what I need," clears up much miscommunication.

The person may not be able or may not choose to give what you want, but you should still express yourself: "I understand that you're having trouble..."

The person may say something like this: "I'm having trouble trusting you. You've let me down before."

"Thanks for telling me straight," you say. "Now, let's talk about it and work on the problem."

Instead of fighting, you're getting the person on your side. Both of you can devote your energies to the problem.

2. You need to share yourself. Allow yourself to become vulnerable and open. You trust; you take risks with others. Sharing with your support person can do so much to relieve your frustrations, anger, exaggerated expectations, anxieties, and depression.

3. You need to define the issues. I urge you to go back into your thought towers. Be as clear as you can about the issues involved. Maybe you're avoiding spiritual issues or responsibility, or you're not willing to face what's going on. Define those things for yourself.

4. You need to be faithful with your exercise and eating plans.

5. You need to be aware of your attitudes and spiritual values. Review chapter 20 on spirituality because your attitude on how you view things and other people can make you feel disappointed, anxious, or at peace. Remember the concepts, and work toward accepting others, giving unconditional love, and exercising more self-discipline.

6. If the issues persist, you may want to get medical and psychiatric evaluations. They may indicate that you have other more severe problems.

You may have financial issues

Many times in life, financial issues become a problem. How do you handle them? Making more money isn't always the answer, and few people can easily find ways to increase their income immediately. Even if you have this opportunity, it may not be the best answer because money is probably not the real issue. Let's look at what you can do for yourself.

1. Don't just wish for things to change. You can say, "I hope this gets better," but that approach doesn't work. You have to make changes. Either decrease your financial needs or make more money. But don't just wish and hope and dream about what would happen if you won a sweepstakes.

2. Incorporate people important to you. Include your spouse, friends, parents—anyone who can help. Get together and say, "I want to talk about how I can get out of this financial hole. Do you have any ideas?"

You may not always want to hear what they tell you. They may strip you bare of some of your illusions. One of them may say to you, "You're a compulsive spender."

I hope you can answer nondefensively with something like this: "I didn't know that. I just knew that every time I needed a reward I'd buy a new toy."

3. Avoiding creditors only makes the situation worse. Contact your creditors and tell them (before the bills are due if possible), "I'm not going to be able to pay my bill." They'll respect you more than after they've called you and tried to track you down, and you say, "Oh, I can't pay it." Instead, level with them: "Look, I'm in trouble. What can we do to work it out?"

Likely, they'll put on the pressure—that's their job.

If you can, give them options: "Three months from now I think I'll be all right, and I'll call you back and let's monitor it. If in three months, I still can't pay, here's what I can do. I can sell my home." Ask them to work with you, and include them as part of the solution instead of looking at them as adversaries.

You owe them money, and they want it. If you can go to them and show a way that you can get it to them by taking a nontraditional approach, they will probably work with you. Do not avoid those issues.

You may say, "I don't have any options here." If you do have an option such as selling something, do it. Don't hang on to a possession just to protect your identity.

You may have to change your life-style temporarily. Or even if it's permanent, you must face your creditors.

4. You need to set up a budget. A budget is useful not only when you have debts to pay but when you want to stay out of debt.

You may suffer from fear and guilt

These two issues are usually evident.

1. Take offensive action. Don't wait for the bombs to strike. Take action first. If you feel guilty about the way you've raised your kids, talk to them. Tell them how guilty you feel.

2. Adopt a forgiving spirit. You need a forgiving spirit—to forgive others and to forgive yourself. Often food dependency has changed the way you think so much that you may want to say, "I've done some things wrong." Instead of feeling bad and letting yourself be consumed with grief and a sense of failure,

forgive yourself. Other people have probably done you wrong, so forgive them.

Go to people you think you've wronged and say, "I've done you wrong. I apologize." Say it directly and simply. If you can go forward with that forgiving spirit, you can work through many, many problems.

♥ ♥ ♥

Vital facts about myself: I forgive those who have wronged me. I forgive myself for the wrongs I have done.

♥ ♥ ♥

You may have other issues

I want you to think about three major things: (1) Don't avoid your conflicts and hassles; hit them head-on; (2) consider your options; and (3) do it now—immediately.

EXERCISE 17:
ISSUES AND GOALS

1. Select up to four issues mentioned in this chapter.
2. Decide on your immediate goal for each issue selected.
3. Write specifically what you will do to reach that immediate goal.

Here is an example. My big issue is finances. My immediate goal is a balanced budget. I will record what I spend so that by the end of this month I can set up a monthly budget with realistic expenditures and know how to handle my finances better.

These are my four issues and the specific action I will take with each one:

1. _____

_____

2. _____

_____

3. _____

_____

4. _____

_____

A FINAL WORD TO YOU

Please continue to work on the principles you have learned in this book. Weight maintenance can be a realistic goal. If you don't ring the bell, you have choices. Focus on eliminating unnecessary bell ringing. Finally, remember to think about the spiritual issues and then HELP YOURSELF TO COMPLETE RECOVERY.